The Best from *Nursing* Magazine

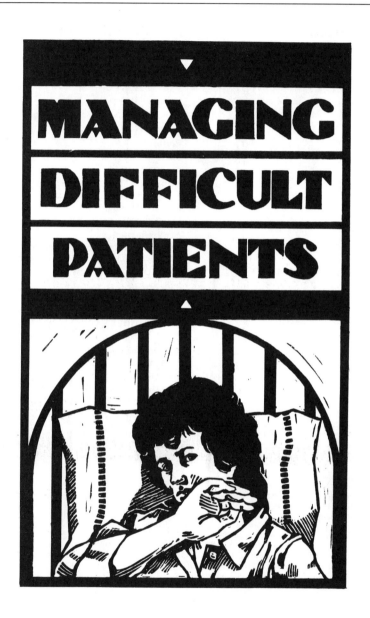

MANAGING DIFFICULT PATIENTS

Springhouse Corporation
Springhouse, Pennsylvania

Staff for this Volume

CLINICAL STAFF

Clinical Director
Barbara McVan, RN

Clinical Editors
Joan E. Mason, RN, EdM
Joanne Patzek DaCunha, RN, BS
Diane Schweisguth, RN, BSN,
CCRN, CEN

PUBLICATION STAFF

Executive Director, Editorial
Stanley Loeb

Executive Director, Creative Services
Jean Robinson

Design
John Hubbard (art director), Stephanie
Peters (associate art director)

Editing
Kathy E. Goldberg

Copy Editing
Katharine G. Tsioulcas (manager), David
Prout (supervisor), Nick Anastasio, Keith
de Pinho, Diane Labus, Doris Weinstock,
Debra Young

Art Production
Robert Perry (manager), Anna Brindisi,
Loretta Caruso, Donald Knauss, Christina
McKinley, Robert Wieder

Typography
David Kosten (manager), Diane Paluba
(assistant manager), Joyce Rossi Biletz,
Brenda Mayer, Brent Rinedoller,
Nancy Wirs

Manufacturing
Deborah Meiris (manager),
T.A. Landis

Project Coordination
Aline S. Miller (supervisor), Elizabeth B.
Kiselev, Laurie Sander

DP-030994

℞ A member of the Reed Elsevier plc group

Library of Congress Cataloging-in-Publication Data
Managing difficult patients.

    Includes index.
    1. Nurse and patient. 2. Nursing—Psychological aspects. 3. Sick—Psychology. I. Springhouse Corporation. [DNLM: 1. Nursing Care—methods. 2. Nursing Care—psychology. 3. Nurse—Patient Relations. 4. Patients—psychology. WY 87 M266]
RT86.3.M36 1988 610.73 88-6672
ISBN 0-87434-136-1

Contents

Contributors

At the time the articles in this book were written, these contributors were affiliated with the following health care facilities.

Patricia Alman, RN
Staff Nurse, Cardiac Care Unit and Medical Intensive Care Unit, Walson Army Hospital, Fort Dix, N.J.

Helen Backus, RN
Staff Nurse, University Hospital, Seattle. Currently, she is Nurse Coordinator of the Osteoporosis Research Study for Dr. Charles H. Chesnut III at the same hospital.

Jane Battersby, RN
This author, who was a member of the *Nursing73* advisory board, wrote her article under a pseudonym. For legal and professional reasons, she wishes to remain anonymous.

Judith Betzold, RN, BS
Staff Nurse, Sequoia Hospital, Redwood City, Calif. Currently, she holds the same position.

Cynthia Blanchard, RN, BSN
Staff Nurse, University Hospital, Seattle.

Karen Jean Bloomfield, RN, BSN
Head Nurse, Neurology, University of Maryland Hospital, Baltimore.

Marie Scott Brown, RN, PhD
Associate Professor, School of Nursing, University of Colorado, Denver. She is currently at Oregon Health Science University, School of Nursing, Portland, Ore.

Ruth Ann Burns, RN, MSN
Clinical Specialist, Psychiatric Unit, Memorial Hospital, Sarasota, Fla.

Lori Carley, RN
Staff Nurse, Cook Children's Medical Center, Fort Worth, Tex. Currently, she holds the same position.

Linda Chitwood, RN, BSN
Staff Nurse, Rush–Presbyterian–St. Luke's Medical Center, Chicago.

Victoria Chura, RN
Staff Nurse, Home Health Service, Community Nursing Services, Johnstown, Pa.

Sue Collier, RN, BSN
Assistant Director of Nursing, Critical Care, St. Vincent Hospital, Indianapolis, Ind.

Rosemarie Selgas Cordes, RN, MSN
Clinical Nurse Specialist, National Cancer Institute, Veterans Administration Medical Center, Washington, D.C.

Florette E. Cramer, RN
Head Nurse, Intermediate Care Unit, Wadsworth Veterans Adminstration Medical Center, Los Angeles.

Marilyn Curran, RN, BSN
Staff Nurse, Veterans Administration West Side Medical Center, Chicago.

Barbara Dossey, RN, CCRN, MS
Staff Nurse, R.H. Dedman Memorial Hospital, Farmers Branch, Tex. Currently, she is Director, Holistic Nursing Consultants, and Director, Bodymind Systems, Dallas.

Joyce Eddy, RN
Research Nurse, National Cancer Institute, Veterans Administration Medical Center, Washington, D.C.

Judith Effken, RN
Head Nurse, Acute Care Unit, Mt. Sinai Hospital, Hartford, Conn.

Lauren Ells, RN
Staff Nurse, Pediatric Unit, University of California Hospital, Los Angeles.

Evelyn Evans, RN, BSN
Staff Nurse, Masonic Cancer Center, University of Minnesota, Minneapolis.

Beverly Z. Faro, RN, MS
Instructor/Clinician II, University of Rochester School of Nursing, Rochester, N.Y. Currently, she is Assistant Professor/Clinician II at the same hospital.

Randi Fuller, RN, BSN
Staff Nurse, Special Care Nursery, Rush–Presbyterian–St. Luke's Medical Center, Chicago.

Mary Ann Gregg, RN, BA
Rehabilitation Specialist, International Rehabilitation Associates, Winter Park, Fla.

Suzanne R. Hesse, RN
Rehabilitation Coordinator, Cooper Hospital–University Medical Center, Camden, N.J. Currently, she is Utilization Review/Quality Assurance Coordinator at the same hospital.

Rosemarie Holmes, RN, BSN
Staff Nurse, Burn Center, Westchester County Medical Center, Valhalla, N.Y. Currently, she is a Clinical Nurse Specialist, Nutrition Support, at the same hospital.

Veronica Hunko, RN
Kings County Hospital Center, New York. Currently, she is Assistant Director of Nursing, Quality Assurance Coordinator at the same hospital.

Marjorie Hurley, RN, BSN
Staff Nurse, Masonic Cancer Center, University of Minnesota, Minneapolis. She is now retired.

Elaine Keniston, RN, BEd
Home Health Aide, Newfound Area Nursing Association, Bristol, N.H. Currently, she is employed by Franklin Regional Hospital, Franklin, N.H.

Patricia M. Koch, RN, BSN
Staff Nurse, Ophthalmology Surgical Unit, George Washington University Hospital, Washington, D.C. Currently, she is Director of Admissions at Hospice of Northern Virginia, Arlington, Va.

Maribell Leavitt, RN, MS
Assistant Professor of Nursing, University of San Francisco School of Nursing, San Francisco.

Lorraine M. Lynn, RN
Staff Nurse, Psychiatric Unit, Valley Hospital, Ridgewood, N.J. Currently, she is self-employed as a freelance writer.

Julie D. Malcolm, RN, BSN
Nursing Skills Laboratory Supervisor, Samaritan College of Nursing, Grand Canyon College, Phoenix, Ariz.

Christine Marek, RN, BSN
Head Nurse, Orthopedic Unit, Hartford Hospital, Hartford, Conn. Currently, she is president of Geriatric Nursing Services, Inc., Glastonbury, Conn.

Lisa Matiak-Mozingo, RN, BSN
Staff Nurse, Emergency Department, Herbert J. Thomas Memorial Hospital, South Charleston, W. Va.

Susan I. Mazique, RN, MPA
Administrative Director of Nursing, Sequoia Hospital, Redwood City, Calif. Currently, she is Associate Administrator at the same hospital.

Anne Meyer-Ruppel, RN, BA
Staff Nurse, Masonic Cancer Center, University of Minnesota, Minneapolis.

Irene M. Misik, RN, BSN
Medical-Surgical Unit, University of Pennsylvania Hospital, Philadelphia.

Regina M. Mueller, RN
Staff Nurse, Surgical Unit, Mercy Hospital, Pittsburgh.

Maureen O'Brien, RN
Chedoke Rehabilitation Center, Chedoke-McMaster Hospitals, Hamilton, Ontario.

Stella K. Oliver, RN
Staff Nurse, Greater Laurel Beltsville Hospital, Laurel, Md. Currently, she is at Prince George's General Hospital and Medical Center, Cheverly, Md.

Karen R. Palermo, RN, BSN
Department of Psychiatry, University Hospital, University of California Medical Center, San Diego.

Martha Petering, RN, MN
Clinical Specialist, Neonatology, Children's Memorial Hospital, Chicago.

Sharon Porter, RN, CCRN, MSN
Clinical Nurse Specialist, Shoal Creek Hospital, Austin, Tex.

Susan Ramage Presley, RN
Washington Regional Medical Center, Coronary Care Unit, Fayetteville, Ark.

Mary Ellen Rebele, RN, BSN
Charge Nurse, Medical Unit, Bloomington Hospital, Bloomington, Ill.

Betty J. Reynolds, RN, MSN
Instructor, Syracuse University School of Nursing, Syracuse, N.Y.

Linda Roberts, RN
Nursing Supervisor, Newfound Area Nursing Association, Bristol, N.H. Currently, she is at Heritage Home Health, Bristol, N.H.

Debbie Casey Royalty, RN, BSN
Intensive Care Unit Staff Nurse, St. Joseph Hospital, Lexington, Ky.

Karen Schaefer, RN, MSN
Assistant Professor, Cedar Crest College, Allentown, Pa. Currently, she is Assistant Professor of Nursing at Allentown College of St. Francis de Sales, Center Valley, Pa.

Carol E. Schreiber, RN
Pottstown Memorial Medical Center, Pottstown, Pa.

Coleen A. Shoemaker, RN, BSN
Staff Nurse, Lehigh Valley Hospital Center, Allentown, Pa. Currently, she is a School Nurse in the Jim Thorpe School District, Jim Thorpe, Pa.

Rita Spillane, RN, BSN
Assistant Professor, College of Nursing, University of Florida, Gainesville.

Kathie Severine Spitz, RN
Staff Nurse, University Hospital, Seattle.

Frances Storlie, RN, MS
Cardiac Nursing Specialist, Emanuel Hospital, Portland, Ore. Currently, she is in the Southwest Washington Health District, Vancouver, Wash.

Dawn A. Taniguchi, RN, BSN
Staff Nurse, Sequoia Hospital, Redwood City, Calif. Currently, she is a Staff Nurse, Medical Personnel Pool, Walnut Creek, Calif.

Carol Tea, RN
Coordinator, Disability Attitude Reassessment Program, Rehabilitation Institute, Detroit.

Mary Jo Tierney, RN, MS
Psychiatric Liaison Clinical Nurse Specialist, Sequoia Hospital, Redwood City, Calif. Currently, she holds the same position.

Elaine A. Tramposch, RN, BSN
Utilization Review Supervisor, Blue Cross/Blue Shield of Greater New York, New York. Currently, she is Administrator, Program Review, Empire Blue Cross and Blue Shield, New York.

Sharon Warlick, RN
Industrial Nurse, Midland Glass Company, Henryetta, Okla. Currently, she is an Executive Secretary at the Oklahoma State Bank and Trust Company, Vinita, Okla.

Margaret Watson, RN
Former Charge Nurse, Sequoia Hospital, Redwood City, Calif.

Diana S. Wilkiemeyer, RN, MS
Private Duty Nurse, Boston. Currently, she is Director of Social Services, Discharge Planning, at Marshall Hale Hospital, San Francisco.

Dolores Zopf, RN
Alternate Team Leader, Imperial Point Hospital, Fort Lauderdale, Fla.

Introduction

Difficult Patient articles have consistently been one of *Nursing's* most successful features. The first article was published in 1973 but is still relevant to nursing practice today.

The natural appeal of these articles comes from their format and content. The format is a story—and we all know that a story is a marvelous teaching device. In the story, the nurse-author gives a first-person account of true incidents that made it unusually difficult to work with a particular patient. The hallmark of the story is the practical solution the nurse uses to resolve the problems encountered in working with this patient.

Although some of the technology mentioned in the articles has changed over the years, the problems each of the difficult patients poses are ones we've all encountered or heard other nurses describe. More important, the solutions used by our colleagues offer each of us a valuable opportunity to change and expand our own nursing practice.

Patricia Nornhold,
Clinical Director
Nursing Magazine

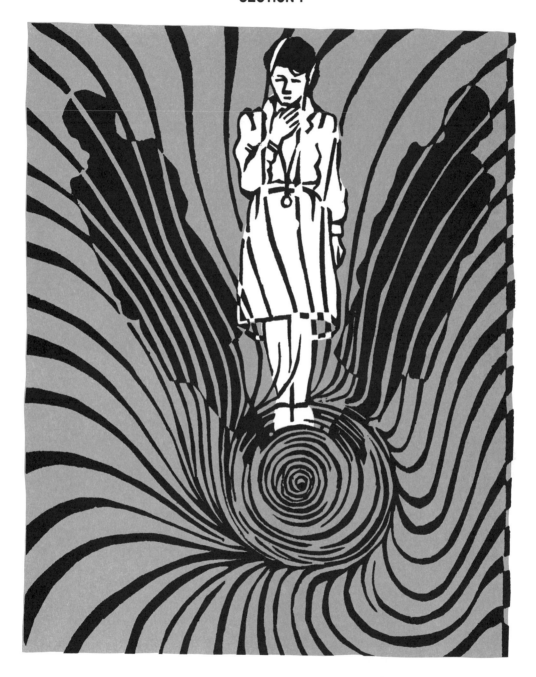

CLINICALLY CHALLENGING PATIENTS

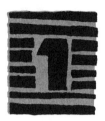

When Just About Everybody Gave Up on Dr. Hyman

ROSEMARIE HOLMES, RN, BSN

For some critically injured patients, the outlook is so dim you have to squint to find a ray of hope. And that's when you tap every ounce of skill and perseverance you have as a nurse—what I like to call nursing persistence. Not that it's easy.

Certainly, it wasn't easy for me during the 4 months Dr. Jay Hyman was a patient in our 10-bed burn unit. A 47-year-old noted marine mammal veterinarian, he'd been in an airplane crash where he'd suffered second- and third-degree burns over 60% of his body.

Alert and able to move his limbs on command when first admitted, he steadily sank into a semi-comatose state like a man sinking into quicksand. He had nasal, maxillary, and frontal sinus fractures, and his nose, right ear, and hair had been badly burned. When he developed a cerebrospinal fluid leak from his nasal cavity, meningitis became a constant threat.

A bronchoscopy upon admission had confirmed his inhalation burns, and since they compromised his respiration, he was immediately placed on a ventilator. His baseline arterial blood gases showed normal oxygen saturation at this time.

To prevent hypovolemic shock, we'd started him on Parkland fluid resuscitation formula and hemodynamic monitoring. His maxillary fracture, coupled with excessive bleeding into his oral cavity, made endotracheal intubation impossible, so the doctor performed a tracheotomy.

Sure, lab tests and clinical procedures tell a lot about a patient, but believe me: Nothing can muffle the shock of seeing somebody who's been seared by high temperatures. Dr. Hyman's face, chest, and arms were pearly white. Most of the rest of his body was blistered and bright red under the silver sulfadiazine. Also, he'd shifted a lot of fluid interstitially in the first 24 hours, making him edematous. Now he looked like a balloon about to pop.

As bad as he looked, I knew his burns could be treated successfully. And after plastic surgery and other surgical intervention, his appearance could be reconstructed.

His head injuries were what really worried me. A neurologic workup yielded negative brain and computerized tomography scan results and clear cerebrospinal fluid upon lumbar puncture. Yet his electroencephalogram findings showed a constant sleep pattern, raising the possibility of irreversible neurologic damage.

As I did a complete head-to-toe assessment, I introduced myself and told him about the burn unit and the kind of treatment he'd be getting, just as I would with any alert patient. I watched closely for some tiny movement of his head, hand, or mouth—some sign that he could hear me. But he didn't move.

Each time I saw him, I continued to talk to Dr. Hyman plainly, slowly, and purposefully. I fully

 But the only sounds in the room other than our voices were the steady beeping of the cardiac monitor and the mechanical swishing of the ventilator. The longer Mrs. Hyman and I tried to get him to respond, and the longer he failed to respond, the more empty and disheartening those sounds became to us.

explained each procedure or treatment before it was done. Also, I taped recent snapshots of his 7-year-old daughter on his bed frame at eye level to remind him of his home life. His wife helped, too. Day after day, she'd sit beside him and talk about their home, friends, and especially their daughter.

But the only sounds in the room other than our voices were the steady beeping of the cardiac monitor and the mechanical swishing of the ventilator. The longer Mrs. Hyman and I tried to get him to respond, and the longer he failed to respond, the

more empty and disheartening those sounds became to us. Each time I walked Mrs. Hyman out of the burn center and then returned alone to Dr. Hyman's room, I grew more worried that he'd never talk or move again.

I was wrong. A week after he was admitted, I was leaving his room after checking his urometer and central venous pressure line when I heard incoherent sounds. Turning, I saw him thrashing about. In a second, his bedclothes were on the floor and he had both legs over the side rails. As I rushed across the room, I spoke to him as calmly as I could: "Dr. Hyman, relax. You're a patient in the burn center, and you must stay in bed."

Next, he grabbed for his intravenous (I.V.) lines and tried to pull them out. I continued to talk to him slowly, reorienting him. Finally, he settled back into bed. His doctor ordered I.V. diazepam (Valium) for anxiety and I.V. morphine for pain.

His agitation had really shaken *me* up. Unfortunately, it was only a prelude.

Two weeks later, he developed septicemia with multiple organisms. At the same time, the progression of antibiotics he was getting reduced his normal body flora, and systemic candidiasis developed. His pneumonia worsened and his blood gas values deteriorated. His PO_2 level dropped to 60 mm Hg...then to 50 mm Hg. We increased the oxygen concentration until we met his respiratory needs.

To improve Dr. Hyman's circulation and mental awareness, we began lifting him out of bed and into a lounge chair for a few minutes daily. Since he was so heavy and limp, transferring him required four nurses. Usually, he'd just sit in the chair, motionless and silent, until we transferred him back to bed.

But one day he surprised us. As we were settling him into the chair, he suddenly became agitated, pushing us aside and vigorously shaking his head back and forth. After we got him back into his bed, I saw his lips moving as if he were trying to speak, so I quickly disconnected his tracheostomy tube from the oxygen tubing and covered the opening by holding a 4x4 gauze pad with my finger. What we heard shocked all of us.

Burn unit delirium, we call it. It's also known as ICU psychosis. Attempting to cope with a catastrophic illness or injury, a patient's imagination

WHEN JUST ABOUT EVERYBODY GAVE UP ON DR. HYMAN

completely takes over. Fantasies become real. Patients are hooked up to so much life-support apparatus they begin to feel like machines themselves. Others—like Dr. Hyman—feel menaced by imaginary beasts. In his delirium, he was talking about iguanas. He said iguanas were climbing on the room walls and ceiling. By now he was really disoriented, pulling at his tubes and dressings, and we had to restrain him to prevent injury. I felt awful, and when his wife didn't visit that afternoon, I felt even worse.

The following day when I saw Mrs. Hyman, I mentioned that we'd missed her the day before. I didn't say a word about her husband's fantasy. "Nurse, can we talk somewhere alone for a minute?" she said. I directed her to the nurses' conference room, where she confessed, "I've been visiting Jay every day for over a month now. Yesterday I woke up and realized I just couldn't come in, because I couldn't bear to see him."

I explained that her reaction seemed perfectly understandable for someone whose husband is balanced precariously between life and death. I also said I was glad she'd come today. She smiled faintly, then looked away.

"There's something else that bothers me," she said. Some years before, when she and her husband had been talking about life and death, he'd said, "If I can't think and act on my own, I don't want to be kept alive by a machine."

Now she had some tough questions for me: Would her husband's survival mean he'd exist only as a custodial patient? Would he be helpless, unable to talk, unable to be part of his family ever again? Suddenly she was crying, and she told me she'd given up all hope of his ever recovering.

That's when my own nursing persistence surfaced. "It's true that his recovery's been slow and painful," I told her. "But his physical condition is improving. Now we've got to encourage him to emerge from the shell he's in."

We returned to his room, and I began to talk to him as if he could understand me. I knew I had to set an example for Mrs. Hyman. And it worked. After a few minutes, she started talking to him, too.

When she left that afternoon, three nurses and I lifted him into the lounge chair again. After 30 minutes, we transferred him back to bed, and I

told Dr. Hyman we'd be moving him into the chair three times every day from then on. Knowing that down under those terrible burns and confusion

 Burn unit delirium, *we call it. It's also known as ICU psychosis. Attempting to cope with a catastrophic illness or injury, a patient's imagination completely takes over. Fantasies become real. Patients are hooked up to so much life-support apparatus they begin to feel like machines themselves. Others—like Dr. Hyman—feel menaced by imaginary beasts.*

there was an intelligent human being, I arranged my care plan to include talking to him appropriately at every contact.

To help raise his level of awareness, I also tried varied auditory and visual stimulation. During the afternoon, I'd tune his radio to a station that played classical music, which he'd always enjoyed. In the evenings I'd switch on the television. Although I didn't notice any response, I thought the familiar sounds of music and television might stimulate Dr. Hyman.

After he'd spent 2 months in the burn center, his complications were under control, and some burn areas were beginning to heal. Finally, his chances for successful skin grafting were improving. But psychologically, a lot of hard work remained ahead for us.

Since Dr. Hyman was a marine veterinarian, I hung photographs of whales on the walls of his room. Also, his young daughter brought in a shark she'd modeled from clay. Every day, I showed Dr. Hyman the shark sculpture and the photograph of his daughter, hoping he'd realize she'd made the gift for him.

A few more weeks passed, and each day I conversed with him by disconnecting his ventilator and plugging the tracheostomy tube. Lying in bed, he rambled incoherently, now and then saying a few words. But he never uttered a logical sentence.

One day, after elevating him on the tilt table, I was taking his blood pressure and looked up at him. Seeing him standing there before me, I suddenly wondered if he might be more willing to communicate now than when he'd been lying in bed.

Tremulously, I disconnected the oxygen source from his tracheostomy tube and covered the opening with a gauze pad as I'd done so many times before. I asked him if he wanted to say anything to me.

No sound.

I asked him again. "Do you want to tell me something, Dr. Hyman?" I waited, feeling my heart beat faster.

Then, in a barely audible voice, he spoke.

"Yes... I've... got... a... few quest... questions... to ask," he said. *My persistence had paid off.* At that moment, I didn't know whether to laugh or cry. I guess I did a little of both.

Two days later, a fenestrated tracheostomy tube was inserted and he started speaking more independently. He also started walking and enjoying solid food. A few weeks later, I found him wearing his favorite bathrobe and talking—haltingly but clearly—to his doctor.

Four months and 2 days after Dr. Hyman first entered our burn center, he was discharged, fully ambulatory, completely alert and oriented. His memory of the critical period of his illness was, he said, "like being in outer space." A long course of therapy and plastic surgery still lay ahead, though.

Now, each time he visits us for physical therapy, I notice an improvement in his appearance *and* his spirits from his cosmetic surgery. He is getting stronger day by day. Next month, he's going to study finback whales off Montauk Point, Long Island.

Maybe some recoveries are truly miraculous— I don't know. But I do know that recoveries like Dr. Hyman's spring from comprehensive assessment and treatment, a flexible care plan, and a lot of plain old nursing persistence.

It Took Ten of Us to Care for Carol — A Very Special New Mother

HELEN BACKUS, RN
CYNTHIA BLANCHARD, RN, BSN
KATHIE SEVERINE SPITZ, RN

Carol was admitted to our unit at approximately 26 weeks intrauterine gestation with a diagnosis of preeclampsia. In the weeks preceding, her baseline blood pressure of 112/70 had risen to 136/92, and she'd developed generalized edema and proteinuria.

Our initial care plan included:
1. Checking her blood pressure, deep-tendon reflexes, and fetal heart tones every 4 hours.
2. Examining her face and extremities for edema.
3. Recording 24-hour fluid intake, urine output, and daily weight.
4. Collecting urine to monitor total protein and creatinine clearance.
5. Requiring strict bed rest with bathroom visits only.

All this would have been fairly routine except for the fact that Carol was 15 years old and had an IQ of 47 according to the Wechsler Scale. That meant she had about as much grasp of her condition as would an 8-year-old child.

Up to 3 months before her admission, Carol had lived at home with her divorced mother and cousin. Her home environment was described as unstable,

and her cousin was suspected of having fathered the baby. Carol had attended a special school for developing prevocational and self-care skills, where she enjoyed handiwork and crafts and had learned to prepare simple meals and tell time. Her teacher described her as a pleasant student, and it was this teacher who suspected Carol's pregnancy and sent her to a gynecologic clinic.

Although abortion was considered, some of Carol's relatives were religiously opposed. Carol's mother had a great deal of difficulty coping with her daughter's pregnancy, and a children's protective service placed Carol in a group home in a nearby city. There, pressured by the change of scene, her pregnancy, and unresolved family conflicts, Carol became uncontrollable and assaultive.

Committed to a psychiatric facility, she was found to be agitated, disoriented, and suffering from hallucinations. Later, she was released and sent to a foster home where she lived fairly quietly until she developed preeclampsia and had to be hospitalized.

When Carol came to us, she seemed shy and frightened. We tried to explain, as simply as we could, why she was in the hospital, what would be done for her, and what her limitations were. We had no way of knowing how much she understood, since she spoke very little.

As the first week went by, Carol became increasingly unhappy and less and less compliant.

 If anyone was going to help Carol, it would have to be us.... She was a threat to herself and her baby.

She refused to stay in bed, and when not closely supervised, she wandered in and out of other patients' rooms, unplugged their electric beds, stole food from the refrigerator, and interrupted procedures. As her restlessness increased, so did her blood pressure, edema, weight, and proteinuria. Often, she refused to save her urine or have blood drawn. Some days, she wouldn't even let anyone check her vital signs. When we tried to insist, she either became belligerent or ran away from us. Naturally, we did all we could to reinforce whatever good behavior she exhibited. But mostly, she wouldn't cooperate enough to let us provide the care we wanted to give.

When we consulted the psychiatric department, they recommended:
• that someone sit with Carol at all times
• that an oral tranquilizer be prescribed
• that we document all medication refusals and instances of threatening or abusive behavior
• that Carol be evaluated by a mental health professional if she became a threat to herself or others.

Round-the-clock sitters (nursing assistants from a temporary agency) allowed us to continually monitor Carol's behavior, but we couldn't see much improvement in it. She still refused most medication, treatment, and tests. She slept only 2 or 3 hours out of every 24, and roamed the unit day and night.

We thought that a family visit and some of her possessions from home might settle Carol a little

and reorient her to reality. But when we called her mother, she was never able to come in. Obviously, if anyone was going to help Carol, it would have to be us. Her potentially life-threatening condition was getting worse and worse. She was a threat to herself and her baby, and the sudden onset of assaultive behavior posed a threat to patients and staff as well. So we called for a mental health professional.

Carol, diagnosed as suffering from acute psychosis, was placed on a 72-hour involuntary hold (which was later extended by a medical continuance) for her own protection and everyone else's. This allowed us to restrain and medicate her as necessary. She didn't like it, of course, but it gave us the chance to structure a long-term, comprehensive care plan that we worked out at a multidisciplinary conference held the next day. We included Carol's three primary nurses, her obstetrician, a psychiatrist, a psychiatric nurse clinician, a hospital social worker, an instructor in behavior modification, and two of the instructor's master's program students.

We agreed to meet once a week thereafter to evaluate our progress and deal with any new problems that might come up. Later meetings would include a nurse from the neonatal intensive care unit, a prenatal nurse clinician, and the nurse coordinator from our unit. Carol's mother was also invited to all the meetings, but she was never able to attend.

We agreed from the beginning that we'd have to maintain a consistent approach, with everyone observing the same rules on every shift. The behavior modification instructor suggested a program of positive and negative reinforcements that were included in Carol's daily nursing plan. This plan would be continuously updated, and by the time of discharge, it was several pages long.

Our first task was to get Carol to take her Navane without force. After that, we believed she'd settle down enough to accept our help. We began by offering Carol the option of taking water or juice with her Navane pill—refusing the pill was *not* one of the options. We promised her a reward if she took the pill and said that we'd medicate her by injection, which she hated, if she refused.

The first time we presented Carol with this choice, she refused Navane by mouth. So we gave her an injection exactly as promised, even though it took *five* people to hold her down. Fortunately, we only had to do this once. The next time, Carol took it by mouth and won her prize. We'd noticed that she loved strawberries, so this was her first reward. Later, we used candy, jewelry, privileges, anything that would provide positive reinforcement for the behavior we needed.

After Carol began taking her Navane regularly, her thought processes improved. She became less paranoid and began to communicate in sentences. Gradually, she came to trust her three primary nurses and her sitters.

Despite these improvements, Carol's restlessness and short memory span created many difficulties. Keeping her in bed with her feet elevated

 Furthermore, she was extremely modest and always bathed or dressed alone with her door closed.... We decided to give Carol only as much generalized information as she could handle before the delivery. That proved to be very little, and we weren't sure she understood that. When the time came, we'd simply have to explain each step as it occurred.

was always a problem. She couldn't complete a given activity without frequent reminders. And we couldn't begin a procedure, leave the room for a moment, come back, and pick up where we'd left off. Carol would have forgotten what we were

doing and would have to have it explained all over again.

These difficulties were never completely resolved, but we could help by maintaining a very firm, consistent schedule. Every morning, we'd wake her, weigh her, and give her her breakfast and medication. Then she'd bathe, and we'd assess her vital signs and preeclamptic checks. After that, we'd get her into a bed or wheelchair with her feet elevated. Afternoon checks were made according to the same pattern. The security of this stable, unvarying routine relaxed Carol and provided reference points to help her remember events.

Any instructions or explanations we gave had to be simple and concrete. We used visual cues whenever we could. Whenever possible, we arranged procedures and activities so they could be completed in one visit. All the while, we gave Carol a lot of feedback on how well she was doing. Praise and rewards were just as important to Carol as any negative reinforcement.

Because of her lower leg edema and elevated blood pressure, Carol absolutely had to remain quiet with her legs elevated. This required a similar behavior modification program. Our goal was to get her off her feet for at least 5 out of every 30 minutes. Taking her to most of her activities in a wheelchair worked well, and often we could persuade her to lie in bed by letting her listen to the record player, color in a coloring book, polish her nails, or listen to a favorite story. After an hour's rest, she could have an outdoor ride in her wheelchair. Sometimes we'd give her another trinket to add to the purse she always carried. Whenever she refused to cooperate, she was confined to her room until she changed her mind.

Gradually, Carol caught on to the system, and her behavior and compliance improved steadily as the weeks went by. Unfortunately, her preeclampsia didn't. We would soon have to start preparing Carol for childbirth. It wouldn't be easy. She was terrified of pain, blood, needles, and any invasive procedure or diagnostic study. Furthermore, she was extremely modest and always bathed or dressed alone with her door closed.

We all agreed that a cesarean section under general anesthesia would produce the least emotional trauma. Even so, we'd still have to prepare Carol for intravenous (I.V.) therapy, the incision, dressings, a Foley catheter, pain, respiratory care, vaginal discharge, and lactating breasts. Because she became upset by any mention of these things, and would probably forget most of what we told her anyway, we decided to give Carol only as much generalized information as she could handle before the delivery. That proved to be very little, and we weren't sure she understood that. When the time came, we'd simply have to explain each step as it occurred.

About a month after her admission, Carol had a large emesis along with increased blood pressure, hyperactive deep-tendon reflexes, and decreased urine output. Then she began to complain of dizziness, and her lab reports indicated that the time had come to put our delivery care plan into action. We prepared Carol as we would any 8-year-old facing major surgery. She got plenty of TLC, the simplest of explanations, and permission to take her teddy bear into the delivery room.

Insertion of the Foley catheter was probably the most traumatizing of the preoperative procedures. Carol trembled and cried as she clung to her teddy bear with one hand and her primary nurse with the other.

After delivering a 2-pound baby girl, Carol awoke with the teddy bear and nurse still at her side. The labor and delivery room nurse had been given a full report on our patient. This included her behavior modification program, since she'd be under their care for the next 24 hours. Because of her preeclampsia, she was placed on a magnesium sulfate I.V. drip after delivery. Pain medications were delivered through the intravenous line rather than by injections that frightened her. A nurse from our unit stayed with her for the first shift, and her regular sitters were with her throughout.

As before, all explanations and directions were kept as simple as possible. We avoided clinical terms whenever we could, substituting "needle" for intravenous, "tube" for Foley catheter, "cut" for incision, "bandage" for dressing, "hurt" for pain, and so on.

Carol returned to our unit a day after delivery and, 4 days later, was eating, walking, and losing weight as her edema diminished.

While Carol's emotional and medical status had presented any number of challenges, her legal status was no less complicated. Though Carol was a ward of the state at the time of hospitalization, was the baby also a ward of the state, or did she belong to Carol?

What would happen to Carol herself? Would she be discharged in custody of her foster mother or her natural mother?

What would happen to her baby?

Because of the baby's undefined legal status, we weren't sure how to handle any relationship between Carol and her daughter. We hesitated to encourage any bonding between them, because we believed the baby would be placed in a foster home. After delivery, we explained to Carol that she'd had a baby girl who was very small and needed special people to care for her. She'd shown little curiosity about her child, and this explanation seemed to satisfy her.

When Carol did visit the neonatal intensive care unit a few days after delivery, she seemed no more interested in her baby than in any of the others, and we still have no idea whether or not Carol related her in any way to her own pregnancy or hospitalization. After she returned to our unit, she never asked to see her baby and visited her only at her mother's insistence.

We're happy to report that today Carol seems well and happy, although unaware that she ever had a baby. We're also happy with the knowledge that imagination, teamwork, and dedication produced an interdisciplinary care plan that saved the lives of two vulnerable young patients.

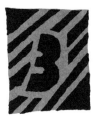

Mrs. Hill Needed More than Caring...and More than a Care Plan

BARBARA DOSSEY, RN, CCRN, MS

We all know how important a caring attitude is. But some patients demand so much attention they stretch our patience to the breaking point. Very often the only way to help them is by combining caring with straight thinking and problem solving. That's what I did with Mrs. Hill, but before I could think straight enough to solve her problems, I had to solve a few of my own.

Mrs. Hill, an independent 69-year-old widow, had been admitted to the hospital while I was on a month's leave. She'd come to the emergency department with shortness of breath and extreme anxiety and was admitted to the medical floor for a workup. Her diagnosis was possible myasthenia gravis, but the doctors felt hypochondriasis played some part, since during the previous year Mrs. Hill had gone from one doctor to another, complaining of "tiredness."

The day after her admission, Mrs. Hill had such trouble breathing that she was transferred to the intensive care unit (ICU). Too hypoxic to speak, she kept writing notes on a legal pad: "I want to stay downstairs. Why am I going to the ICU?"

Mrs. Hill was intubated and put on a BEAR 1 ventilator. When attempts to wean her were unsuccessful, the doctors did a tracheotomy. But the staff suspected that Mrs. Hill didn't need the ventilator and that her dependency was emotional.

For one thing, although she had shown signs of diaphragmatic paralysis at first, it was only temporary. For another, her behavior was almost stereotypical of severe hypochondria. Mrs. Hill had a thousand unrelated complaints, which she would write out on a yellow legal pad. She also had an incredible amount of medical information and misinformation. And she was forever writing things like "Don't leave me, I'm dying!"

Nothing the nurses or doctors could say eased her fear. And although they would take her off the ventilator for a while, they couldn't keep her off it. She was so demanding of the nurses that none of them wanted to be assigned to her for more than a few days at a time.

The nurses' job was made even harder by the fact that, because of Mrs. Hill's varied complications, several different specialists—including a neurologist, an endocrinologist, and a cardiologist—were writing often-conflicting orders for her.

Unfortunately, none of the doctors could come up with a definite diagnosis. Add to this the fact that Mrs. Hill had no outside source of emotional support. A 75-year-old aunt visited her just twice, finally snorting to the nurses as she left: "She's a hypochondriac." Indeed, Mrs. Hill had apparently given up on herself, because she'd made up her mind to sell her house and go into a nursing home.

I came back to the hospital on Mrs. Hill's 29th day, and were the other nurses ever glad to see me. Since I *like* the challenge of working with difficult patients, the other nurses were eager to have me take my turn with Mrs. Hill. But it didn't take me long to realize that this woman could make me a wreck.

After hearing report and reading the previous week's nurses' notes, I made a nursing care plan using nursing diagnoses. Then I went to meet Mrs. Hill. She was asleep, with the ventilator humming. Her hair was in disarray, her eyes were half open, and a nasogastric tube dangled from one nostril. There were sores at the sides of her mouth from her continual use of a tonsil suction. The nurses had let Mrs. Hill suction her mouth to try to get her involved in her own treatment, but the plan had backfired. Now Mrs. Hill wouldn't swallow her saliva.

One of the respiratory therapists was in the room, and I asked him about the ventilator and pulmonary orders. Although we were saying nothing Mrs. Hill shouldn't hear, I glanced over occasionally to make sure she was still asleep. Apparently so. But the second the therapist left, Mrs. Hill began rattling the bedrail. Then she began writing on her yellow pad. She had beautiful penmanship—cursive script that was almost artwork. But you needed the patience of a saint because she took forever to write one sentence. "Who," she wrote, "did you say you were?"

I answered, realizing she'd awakened some time during my conversation. Then came a series of other questions: "Are you a new nurse? Are you sure you know how the ventilator works? Why were you asking so many questions about it?"

After this came a string of demands that had me running all over and, in between, my pulses hammering. I had to stand there while Mrs. Hill slowly wrote out what else she had in mind for me. After 3 hours (and it was only 10 a.m.), I knew I had to take a break. I asked one of the other nurses to relieve me, and she said "sure," with a look of real sympathy on her face.

A lot of nurses don't seem to realize that their salaries cover a daily 15- or 30-minute break. So they just grab a fast cup of coffee and hurry back to work. Well, you're no good to your patients if you're no good to yourself. You should use your break to back off from the situation, to sit down and relax. When I'm up against tensions, I use my breaks to do relaxation exercises.

I went into an empty patient room and, sitting there, realized I was breathing irregularly and the back of my neck was in knots. The technique I use—which anyone can learn—is from Herbert Benson's book, *The Relaxation Response*. As you rhythmically breathe in and out, you concentrate on relaxing different sets of localized muscles. I started by relaxing my head, jaw, and neck muscles, trying to free my mind of all the nursing care I had to do.

Relaxed, I was able to see that I'd deserted holistic nursing. Instead of treating Mrs. Hill as a whole person, I'd fallen into the old trap of simply treating sick organ systems.

Mrs. Hill had really begun to get me angry, and the angrier I got, the harder I concentrated on the *tasks* involved, pushing the human being further into the background. Getting in touch with my own stress also made me aware that one cause of Mrs. Hill's behavior was that she didn't see herself as participating in her own care. I now saw her in a different way, as someone I cared for tremendously—though nothing had changed but *me*.

Back in Mrs. Hill's room, sitting by her bed with my hand on her arm, I said, "I've just spent 3 exhausting hours with you. I want you to participate with me in helping you. The only way you can get well is if you start trying."

She looked at me, smiling slightly. Then she wrote, "I'll try. What do you want me to do?" I told her I wanted to make a contract with her in which we would both go task by task, completing each task before starting another. She wrote, "Okay," but within 5 minutes she was as demanding and manipulative as before. When I brought it to her attention that she wasn't keeping our contract, she acted mad—but she did try a little.

I knew that 29 days of that kind of behavior couldn't be changed in a day. But based on what I knew about Mrs. Hill, I was optimistic that we could work together successfully.

A few years ago I'd developed a psychosocial assessment tool that I call PERSON, and it's proven quite successful for me. I used it to identify the following in Mrs. Hill:

• *Personal* strengths—she was the most alert ventilator patient I'd ever cared for; she wrote clear, descriptive notes; nothing got by her;

• *Emotional* state—severe anxiety; she was afraid to fall asleep for fear she'd stop breathing;

• *Response* to stress—manipulation and depression;

• *Support* systems—just the staff, most of whom had about given up on her;

• *Optimal* health goal—none that I knew of, since I couldn't get her to express any motive for getting well;

• *Nexus,* the body-mind connection. She believed she was ill, therefore she was.

But before I left that afternoon, Mrs. Hill wrote something I wasn't quite sure how to take. "You're not going to take care of me tomorrow, are you?" I didn't know whether she didn't *want* me to, or was afraid I wouldn't. I said, "I sure hope I can."

What she wrote next made everything even more cryptic. "Maybe I dreamed it, but I think I was off of this ventilator for a couple hours last week."

Before leaving the hospital, I asked one of the respiratory therapists about this, and he said that Mrs. Hill *had* been off the ventilator for 4 hours. But because she insisted on going back on the ventilator, the staff had become even more discouraged. However, it had the opposite effect on me. I felt that by giving me this information Mrs. Hill might be saying, "I was off the ventilator. Help me again."

The next day, after a discussion with the staff, I spoke with Mrs. Hill about a new care plan she could participate in. Phrasing each idea carefully, I asked her what I could do then to help her feel better. She wrote, "Could you wash my hair?"

I said I'd be glad to and then told her some things we could do together to also make her feel better. She could try to swallow on her own so she wouldn't need the tonsil suction, and she could start eating soft foods so we could eventually do away with the nasogastric tube. She could also move to a new room, where she could look at the street rather than the ICU corridor; could see traffic, and people, and *life*. And she could try to *walk* part way to her new room without the ventilator. Once there, we would work to get her off the ventilator for good.

I stood there anxiously as Mrs. Hill began writing. My heart leaped as I read: "You think I can do all that?" "Not alone," I said. "We'll all work together." Again, that slow, beautiful writing. It said simply: "I'll try."

That morning, I washed and dried Mrs. Hill's hair. Then I lifted the suction tube from her mouth and asked her to swallow. She did—hesitantly at first, then again. She did it several more times, then smiled.

Now that she knew she could swallow, she realized she could also eat, and I told her we'd give her five small meals a day.

"What soft food would you like right now?" I asked.

"A scrambled egg turned over twice," Mrs. Hill wrote.

That sounded reasonable, so I went to the dietary department with Mrs. Hill's request. Fifteen minutes later, I was back in her room. I helped her eat the egg—the first solid food she'd had in 2 weeks—and she beamed with pleasure.

A few hours later, we were ready to transfer Mrs. Hill to her new room. One of the other nurses had already moved Mrs. Hill's possessions; another had done all the necessary paperwork. Two nurses and two respiratory therapists were with me in the room, all of us linked by a sense of excitement.

It was now time to unhook Mrs. Hill from the ventilator. It was on a low setting, so Mrs. Hill was doing much of her own breathing. She held onto the chief respiratory therapist's and my arms, and we walked the *whole* distance to her new room. Though we had a wheelchair ready, Mrs. Hill didn't even look at it. As she eased back into her new bed, where she was hooked up again to the ventilator, she looked as proud of herself as we were of her.

Shortly afterward, the pulmonary specialist, the respiratory therapists, and I got together to make plans to wean Mrs. Hill from the ventilator. But first, we had to see that she got more sleep. She'd had so many orders from different doctors, and so many things were being done for her day and night, that she was exhausted and perhaps becoming disoriented from lack of sleep.

We wanted to be sure she got 90 minutes of uninterrupted sleep between treatments, so we hung a big notepad on her door and printed a new sign every 90 minutes, telling everyone to stay out until such-and-such a time.

Believe it or not, Mrs. Hill was off the ventilator within 24 hours. And a couple weeks later she was transferred to a medical floor.

I had been assigned to Mrs. Hill for just 2 days, but her impact on me and on the other nurses in the ICU was so great that I felt this was a case—no, a *person*—that could help all nurses. I organized a nursing grand rounds, and got permission from Mrs. Hill to videotape an interview with her on her experience in the ICU.

I started off by asking her what she remembered about me and what, if anything, I'd done that had helped her. Her response was: "I thought the head nurse sent you in as the motivator to get me well. Isn't that your title—'motivator'?"

"No. My title is staff RN."

"I thought all along it was motivator," she said. "You washed my hair, you touched me like you cared, you made me feel I could help myself."

I would pop in on Mrs. Hill now and then on the medical floor, and from what I saw and heard, quite a transformation took place. No, not so much in Mrs. Hill. She remained demanding—she had certain expectations. Rather, the transformation was in the *nurses*. Understanding Mrs. Hill better, they began to like her, to look on her in a different way so her demands didn't come across as demands.

Mrs. Hill did go to a nursing home after she left the hospital, but then she returned to her own home. A year later, she was admitted to another hospital and diagnosed as having myasthenia gravis. So she'd probably had early symptoms while she was at our hospital.

Mrs. Hill didn't teach me to be *caring*—I think I've always been that. And she didn't teach me to dig in and solve problems—I think I knew how to do that before. Rather, she reminded me—and how often we need reminding—of how important it is to combine the two.

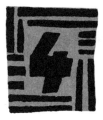

A Lesson in Living

LINDA CHITWOOD, RN, BSN

Caring for a dying newborn is a demanding, draining responsibility that few professionals would expect to pass on to unskilled, impoverished parents. Nonetheless, when Connie's parents asked for that responsibility, it became my job to prepare them for the task.

Connie Cook, born on Valentine's Day in a rural community hospital, was the first child of a poor, barely literate, teenage mother and her older, estranged husband. At 8 pounds (3.6 kg), 21 inches (52.5 cm), Connie looked like a normal baby. Tragically, however, she'd been severely asphyxiated at birth. Even though she was resuscitated in the delivery room, the severity of the perinatal asphyxia and the intensity of the neurologic damage left no hope at all.

Two hours after her birth, Connie was admitted in critical condition to our regional neonatal intensive care unit. We began mechanical ventilation and inserted an umbilical artery catheter to administer fluids and draw blood samples. Continuous monitoring of her heart rate, respiration, and temperature was also started.

At 6 hours of age, Connie went into seizures caused by the cerebral edema often seen in asphyxiated infants. Intravenous phenobarbital and phenytoin (Dilantin) were tried without success. Even paraldehyde gave little control, and neurologists could offer no alternatives. Then, at 10 hours of age, Connie began breathing on her own, and the seizures decreased. By 18 hours, she was extubated and breathing adequately without mechanical ventilation. For the time being, we would offer life-supporting measures until the cerebral edema that accompanied the asphyxia subsided and a more accurate assessment of her status could be made. Unfortunately, time brought little, if any, change in Connie's condition. Notations like "grossly abnormal EEG... limited life expectancy...poor prognosis" still glared up from the pages of her chart.

Our unit had just begun primary nursing, and I warily signed on as Connie's primary nurse. After conferring with her doctor and social worker, I went to work on a care plan. Our first goal was to maintain a patent airway. An Ambu bag, mask, oxygen, and suctioning equipment were kept at her bedside. Unable to swallow or suck, Connie had copious, thick secretions that had to be suctioned from her nasopharynx and oropharynx as often as 10 to 12 times per 8-hour shift. We tried increasing her fluid intake to decrease the viscosity of her secretions, but that didn't help much at all.

Our second goal was to maintain an adequate fluid and electrolyte balance. At first, Connie received total parenteral nutrition (TPN) through a peripheral vein. Later, we gradually introduced infant formula through a continuous nasogastric tube drip. More than a week passed before she was able to tolerate these feedings, then we gradually discontinued TPN.

Brain damage had left Connie with no sucking reflex at all. Every day, a physical therapist would run a nipple around the edges of Connie's lips, then on her lips, then in and out of her mouth. All to no avail. Eventually, Connie would have to have a gastrostomy. This at least would let us get formula straight into her stomach and lessen the risk of aspiration, a common threat to infants with seizure disorders.

Seizure control was our third goal, but we never really attained it. In fact, we could provide little more than routine seizure care—rolling her on her side and holding her gently to keep her from hurting herself. Despite therapeutic levels of phenobarbital and Dilantin, Connie still had seizures with trembling extremities, bradycardia, cyanosis, and occasional apnea. Eventually one of the seizures would prove fatal. Until then we could only maintain life and wait for the inevitable.

Several days after Connie's admission, I realized that my care plan needed another goal—along with caring for Connie, I was going to have to meet her parents' needs as well. Married only 8 months, they'd separated a week before Connie's birth. When Connie's father, Clyde, learned of her condition, he borrowed a car and drove the 50 miles (80 km) to our center. Overwhelmed by the sight of his helpless child, he slumped into a chair by her bedside, buried his head in his hands, and wept. A social worker gently consoled and counseled him, but he still seemed stunned and bewildered when he left. Frankly, few of us expected to see him again. We'd all seen parents of children like this—they take one horrified look and can never bring themselves to return.

Several days later, Clyde surprised us with a second visit. He'd pulled himself together and was ready to discuss his daughter's future. The social worker, doctor, and I gave him our views as frankly as we could. Connie's condition had been thoroughly evaluated by several specialists, and we believed that no heroic measures could improve the quality of her life.

At the end of a grim and taxing encounter for all of us, Clyde agreed to go home and discuss the situation with Connie's mother.

The next day, Clyde returned with his wife, Annie, a shy, timid teenager. They had talked through the night, Clyde said, and they'd finally come to a decision.

"We want Connie home with us. If she is going to die, let her die in our home, where she belongs. She's our child."

We'd rarely been able to send babies like this home with their parents, and Connie was an especially difficult patient to care for—even in a hospital. She had to be suctioned at least every hour. She vomited frequently. She needed constant attention. She responded to touching and manipulation with coarse crowing or shrill crying. Even a well-organized, financially secure family would find caring for a child like Connie a demanding, heartbreaking job. The Cooks' circumstances made it seem impossible.

Virtually penniless, they lived in a clapboard shack in the middle of a field. They had fresh well water and electricity, but that was it. With no heating or cooling system, the shack was alternately drafty and stuffy. There was no refrigerator to keep formula, no stove to heat it, and no telephone to call for help. Further, even if they could handle the task, was it fair to let Clyde and Annie take their baby home only to wake up some morning and find her dead?

But, difficult or not, fair or not, this was what the Cooks wanted. They convinced us of that. So returning Connie to her family became the fourth goal of our nursing care plan.

First of all, we'd have to provide a way for Connie to be fed. She couldn't take anything by mouth because she couldn't suck. So we transferred her to a nearby children's hospital for a gastrostomy tube insertion. She tolerated the surgery well and was all ready to restart feedings when we met an obstacle none of my discharge planning had foreseen. The staff doctor assigned to Connie refused to have her readmitted to our unit after her surgery.

"We're not a surgical unit," he argued. "Let the other hospital do the discharge teaching and send her home from there. She doesn't need intensive care any more, and it might be months

 Even a well-organized, financially secure family would find caring for a child like Connie a demanding, heartbreaking job. The Cooks' circumstances made it seem impossible. Virtually penniless, they lived in a clapboard shack in the middle of a field. They had fresh well water and electricity, but that was it.

before we could send her home."

Having had little success in the past with discharging similar infants to their homes, he felt we had no chance with this one, especially in light of her social situation.

I could see his point, but I couldn't agree. We'd already established a hard-won rapport with the Cooks, and I believed asking them to start new relationships with new doctors, new nurses, and new social workers would be disastrous. I just wasn't sure they could do it. It took me several conferences to get my point across, but Connie was readmitted to our unit the next day. Three days later, she was on full feedings, and her parents were ready for discharge teaching.

Getting Connie home would involve the com-

bined efforts of social services, physical therapy, medicine, and nursing.

Our plan was to have Annie provide total care for Connie while she was in the unit. We would demonstrate all the skills, and Annie would practice them until she could successfully return the demonstration.

Before Annie could take her daughter home, she'd have to learn to:
1. Clear her airway with a suction catheter or bulb syringe.
2. Feed her through a gastrostomy tube and care for the site.
3. Give her medications.
4. Carry out routine baby care, including diapering, bathing, safety, and positioning.
5. Care for Connie during her seizures.
6. Carry out range-of-motion exercises.

Clyde had planned to come with Annie and learn these skills, but he'd just found a job, and the money was badly needed. So Annie came alone, prepared to stay as long as it would take to learn to care for her baby.

The day she arrived, I sat down with her full of hope and excited about the possibilities. It was probably a blessing that I didn't know what I was getting into.

After carefully explaining to Annie that she should feed the baby every 3 hours and medicate her 3 times a day, I asked her how often she would feed and medicate Connie.

"I feed her 3 times a day, and give her medicine every 3 hours," she answered proudly with a broad smile.

Although I felt Annie could learn, it wasn't going to be easy. First of all, she obviously had trouble concentrating in the middle of a busy, 15-bed intensive care unit. So I moved Connie and Annie to a far corner of the unit behind privacy screens, and pretty soon we were in business.

Annie was a simple, inexperienced girl, but with clear instructions and repeated demonstrations, she could catch on. I made my instructions relate to life as she saw it—not as I did. For example, I finally straightened out the medication schedule by telling her to medicate Connie when the sun came up, when it went down, and in the middle of the night. I didn't try for exactitude.

We went over and over everything from bathing

to suctioning. For the latter, we used either a bulb syringe or a straight catheter attached to a 35-cc syringe with traction applied to the barrel to create suction. Annie picked up suctioning very quickly and turned out to be very alert to the baby's needs. In fact, she proved to be surprisingly adept at all the physical skills needed to care for Connie. She kept the gastrostomy tube as clean as any professional. When it came to routine baby care, even though she had to mix powdered formula for every feeding since there was no refrigerator at home, you'd think she'd been a mother all her life.

I'd lined up two very tolerant and patient nurses to help Annie on the 3-to-11 and 11-to-7 shifts in my absence, and I went home that afternoon feeling we'd made a pretty good start. When I arrived at 6 a.m. the next day, Annie said, "It's almost time to give her her medications and feed her, but I think she needs to be suctioned first."

"A+, Annie," I said. We'd made an even better start than I'd hoped for.

A few days later, Clyde paid a friend to drive him to the center to pick up his family. Clutched in his big hand was a tiny pink dress for his daughter to wear home. So Connie was discharged to a life-style few of us can even imagine, her crib a bureau drawer padded with worn blankets. But the Cooks were a family again, and Connie was home with them as they wished.

Then one cold and bleak morning, as we'd all expected, the Cooks awoke to find that their baby had died quietly during the night.

Several months after Connie's death, I met the doctor who'd been her resident. I told him how we'd obtained a gastrostomy tube, how we taught her parents to care for her, how she'd been discharged to her parents' home, and finally how she had died.

"What? She died!" he exclaimed. "Why, I thought you were going to tell me she'd been saved and was doing well today." Frowning, he turned abruptly and stalked off.

For most medical people, success means saving lives. By those standards, nursing Connie and her parents should have been an exercise in failure. Yet I think this painful experience taught me as much about the meaning and purpose of nursing as any I've had. Patients and their families have rights and needs that must be met, regardless of the outcome of the case. If we nurses don't meet them, who will?

Cletus – A Man with Just Too Many Problems

SUZANNE R. HESSE, RN

We nurses hear a lot about considering the whole patient and trying to honor his wishes. But faced with a mercurial, violent, irresponsible patient, the only guidelines available may be the ones you work out for yourselves. So I learned from Cletus.

Cletus had arrived in our Emergency Room directly from the county jail where he was being held on a theft charge. This 20-year-old Black youth had a long acquaintance with trouble. A known drug addict, former convict, former mental patient, Cletus had behaved so wildly in jail, he'd been placed in solitary. There, he set fire to his mattress, was accidentally caught in the flames, and received second- and third-degree burns on the face, neck, legs and feet, totaling 40 to 50% of the body.

After Emergency Room treatment, he was ordered to Intensive Care, then Burn Therapy, and approximately 2 months after admission, transferred to our department, Rehabilitation.

Just reading the doctors' and nurses' progress notes gave us some idea of what to expect. On the fifth day, he had started to become uncooperative: "Doesn't want Foley out. Won't get out of bed.

At times is abusively loud." He refused outright to go to Hubbard tank. He was given to arguing and laughing loudly with one non-existent "Maxie"; he shouted profanities at imaginary voices in the hall.

On the tenth day, a doctor active in a community drug program was called in to evaluate the patient. His findings were subclinical behavior disturbance prior to the accident and, with the history of hard drug use, perhaps some deterioration of cerebral function enhanced by electroyte imbalance.

This, then, was the patient we awaited.

The physiatrist's program for correcting Cletus' arm and leg contractures was very explicit: bedside range-of-motion exercises for all joints; frequent turning on the CircOlectric bed; Hubbard tank at 90 degrees for 30 minutes twice a day; and occupational therapy for function and range of motion.

Less clear was just how we were supposed to get Cletus to do these things.

In our staff discussion, we reviewed the patient's history of doing only what he wanted—when he wanted to do it. Such behavior can only result in incomplete therapy and slow healing. So we decided that for the patient's own benefit all treatments would be carried out—regardless of his objections.

And object, Cletus did.

When he was taken to the Hubbard tank, the Betadine and sloughed-off skin floating in the water didn't deter him from taking mouthfuls and spitting it on anyone he could reach.

When it came time to get him on his feet, he would just swing on the arms of those trying to stand him up.

He bit two therapists.

But we were determined to maintain the schedule. When it came time for whirlpool, we simply told him that we were going to put him on the stretcher and the attendant would take him to Physical Therapy. After a few rounds of protest (which he always seemed to need) he went to PT.

The same system worked with turning him on the CircOlectric. If his comments seemed reasonable at all—"put a pillow (or bath blanket) at my feet"... "put a drawsheet over my stomach"... "position me while I'm on my stomach"—we would give them a try. In this way, we gave him some control over the turning while we maintained control over the schedule.

We tried to give immediate attention to any reasonable request. When he complained about the pressure of sheets on his toes and heels and the standard bed cradle would not fit the CircOlectric, we improvised a tunnel from a sturdy cardboard box to keep the covers off this painfully burnt area.

Cletus soon threw himself out of the CircOlectric bed, however, and had to be put in a regular hospital bed with guard rails.

And, when it came to throwing, Cletus didn't stop with himself.

The hollering, vulgarity and recalcitrance we had been prepared for. What we hadn't foreseen was the radio hurtling out into the hallway. Or the pitchers being crashed to the ground. Or the foodstuffs and clothing thrown about.

If this was wearing on the staff, and it was, you can imagine how it affected the sick. They were fatigued by the noise and frightened by the violence. And, rightly, they complained.

Ideally, we should have put Cletus in a private room on a floor especially designated for violent patients. In our hospital, this wasn't possible, so we worked around it as best we could. We put Cletus in a room by himself and moved patients who would be least affected (comatose or other noisy patients) into adjoining rooms.

This helped a little, but not much.

The one thing that gave us heart was seeing that the enforced treatments and tight control of the situation was working. After only a few days of Hubbard tank, better healing started because dead, sloughing skin and excess dry ointment were removed and granulation became more rapid. Cletus *was* healing and the day finally came when he began to request whirlpool!

If, at one point, Cletus with his schizophrenia, heroin addiction and painful burns seemed like the biblical Job beset with modern plagues, perhaps we should have been alert for further burdens destined his way.

But we weren't. And they came from the last quarter we would have expected: his family and friends.

It soon was apparent that the patient became noticeably more irrational after he had had visitors. We felt that some of his friends were supplying him with drugs other than the medication ordered by the physician. The medical and nursing staff then decided to restrict visitors to the immediate family.

Unfortunately, this didn't bring much of an improvement. Every patient, perhaps especially a burn patient, needs to feel good support, understanding, and encouragement from a relative or friend. Those closest to the patient must encourage him to work with the staff. When we approached Cletus' father, however, he proved to be unreliable and not really interested, saying that his estranged wife and son were just alike and that he couldn't do anything with either of them.

Cletus' mother, an attractive working woman who visited her son regularly, brought him everything he requested—food, a radio, TV. Unfortunately, they frequently had loud arguments over very minor things, and at one point Cletus cut his wrists in her presence.

It was this need for unrelenting vigilance that was so hard on the staff.

We realized, for example, that even such a trying patient as Cletus needs some companionship and we would wheel him to the solarium to give him some contact with others. Predictably, he disturbed them but just as he appeared to be adjusting some, the inhalation therapist who went to the solarium to treat another patient found two syringes missing from her cart. She called the charge nurse who found them tucked in Cletus' pajama waistband.

He was also very graphic in commenting on staff members who appealed to him physically and we had to be one step ahead of his quick hands. We had a policy of not showing horror, shock or amusement when this happened. We simply removed his hands and made no further reference to such behavior.

Harder to ignore was our own morale. Staff spirit and patience reaches the lowest level when a patient who is abusive, vulgar, and violent is also long-term. We discussed this, and when we realized there were times we were starting to dread our work day, we decided to assign a different staff member to the patient daily. We emphasized that whoever was responsible for Cletus that day had to be alert to the mood swings and hostility and be capable of managing whatever arises. It was important not to use a staff member whom Cletus could intimidate or manipulate.

In the final stages of Cletus' hospitalization, it seemed inevitable that our plans for his long-term care and placement should develop all kinds of snags. The state vocation rehabilitation assistance we applied for was cancelled because of Cletus' psychiatric problems and unlikelihood of a good prognosis.

Commitment papers to a state psychiatric hospital were started, but the mother not only refused to sign but threatened a suit against the hospital. So the social service withdrew papers for an involuntary commitment.

After weeks of working on placement, the decision was made to transfer Cletus to a county hospital. This was clearly not the best possible solution. In our hospital, we were able to protect our other patients from abuse and possible physical harm. But most county hospitals are made up of open wards where Cletus would pose a serious problem. The county hospital, however, also contained a large psychiatric facility and the psychiatrist felt that once the patient was in the institution, it would be easier to transfer him from one department to another.

As it turned out, Cletus lasted exactly 2 days in the county hospital before transfer to a state psychiatric facility.

Cletus had been with us 4 months and 20 days. When he left, his burns were healed; he walked; fed himself; was continent; and with the exception of right wrist and hand contractures, was in general, physically improved. The one thing that hadn't changed was his irrational abusive behavior.

If there is one thing we learned from this case, it's that with a multi-problemed, irresponsible patient like Cletus, there is no prepared script. You must innovate. The entire staff must join together to evaluate the situation and formulate a plan of action. And then stick to it!

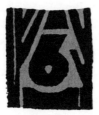

Pathology–Not Personality–Caused Our Problems with Leon

PATRICIA M. KOCH, RN

Leon Bradley, a 25-year-old government clerk, had such poor vision that he couldn't read an eye chart. In fact, he could barely count the fingers on a hand held 12 inches (30 cm) in front of his face.

The major cause of his ocular degeneration and visual impairment was juvenile-onset diabetes mellitus, and he was admitted to our 18-bed eye surgery unit in late summer for a cataract extraction from the right eye. Two weeks later, he returned for a tricky pars plana vitrectomy of the left eye to correct a severe vitreous hemorrhage that had not resolved in the previous 6 months.

With his smooth-as-molasses West Virginia accent and clean-cut good looks, Leon seemed more like a boy than a man to us. He radiated friendliness, but his fellow patients—most of whom were 50 years older than he—could offer him little companionship.

His roommate was a cheerful and intelligent man. But at 80 years old, his own failed eyesight and faulty hearing made him an unlikely companion. Across the hall, a 72-year-old woman patient rambled on day and night—about her health, her intense discomfort, and her sister, who'd recently died. Her long monologues grated on everyone's nerves, and one evening when Leon called me into his room, I thought for sure he would insist, as other patients had, that we sedate the woman to keep her quiet. But Leon just smiled and politely asked me to shut his door so he could get some sleep.

We tried to make Leon feel less lonely by looking in on him several times each shift, and since most of us were close in age to Leon, these daily meetings became a pleasant change of pace for us, too. We also stretched official visiting hours to give Leon's family and friends—especially his girlfriend—a chance to visit.

For practical reasons, Leon was classified as "Treat As Blind" (TAB) on his chart, patient-care Kardex, and in all our verbal reports. A TAB label means the patient should be oriented to the unit when he's admitted and reoriented p.r.n.

Here's how we do that. We talk and "feel" him around his room, counting steps to the bathroom, while fixing relative placement of furniture, closets, telephone, and call bell.

Furniture and patient belongings are always left

in agreed-upon places, since slight shift in placement can easily cause injury or embarrassment. We also position all doors either completely open or completely closed. Few things are more harmful to a blind patient (who fans ahead with his hands as he walks) than the narrow, sharp edge of a half-open door.

We also help the patient with his daily activities, including personal hygiene, meal selection, and eating. A bath station is set up by placing a chair at the sink or by bringing the basin to the overbed table. We also routinely wash the patient's back and feet, assisting with special diabetic foot care. Although most postoperative patients on our unit are forbidden to shave or shampoo, we help those who are allowed.

When it comes to mealtimes, we read the menu to the patient and circle his favorite foods. For setting up meal trays, we use the clock-dial system, placing specific foods at "12 o'clock" or "3 o'clock" positions, and so on. Beverages are always set at the back of the tray to prevent spills, and hot drinks are never filled to the top of the cups. Since we believe it's better for a patient to feed himself even if he makes a little mess, we provide a Chux, towel, or extra gown in addition to his paper napkin.

"Nothing's more frightening than hearing *only* footsteps," Leon told us once. So we always made a point of saying "Hello" when we entered his room and "Good bye, Leon" when we left. Verbal cues are also important before touching a blind patient. A touch coming out of nowhere can be terrifying, no matter how soothing its intent.

Finally, all TAB patients like Leon are given diversions, including Talking Books (both records and cassettes), as well as earplug hookups to the local "Ear" radio station, which reads newspapers and magazines to the visually handicapped. We encourage all TAB patients to use battery-operated radios; and we place telephones within easy reach.

With Leon, we tried to carry out all TAB procedures as faithfully as possible and at the same time respect his privacy and independence. Being flexible helped. For example, we postponed Leon's daily bath and linen change when his brother was coming to visit because he wanted to help with Leon's care. Such family involvement strengthened Leon's will to recover.

Leon's postoperative eye care was a series of potential crises. For the first 3 days after the vitrectomy, he was forced to lie flat on his stomach in bed with his face resting between two pillows. He had to maintain that difficult position to ensure that the air bubble, which had been injected into his left eye, floated up and held the retina in place. After a few days, the hydrostatic pressure of the balanced salt solution, BSS (a saline solution with electrolytes added), used to replace his aqueous humor would stabilize. During those long 72 hours, Leon could get up only for 30-minute meal periods and one bowel movement daily. Still, even those activities had to be done with his head held down.

To reduce Leon's discomfort and edema, we provided him with ice-water compresses to the forehead and eyes every hour. When he complained of nasal congestion and sinus headache as well as eye pain, we offered him Sudafed, 30 mg, P.O., every 4 to 6 hours, along with two acetaminophen with codeine (Tylenol #3) tablets. To stop his tissues from desiccating from those medications, we gave him as many sugar-free drinks as he wanted.

Included in his postoperative eye care were two sets of medications, one set for each eye. To prevent medication errors and save time, we fixed separate plastic medication boxes for the right eye (OD) and the left eye (OS). By convention, the right eye is always taken care of first. We labeled each box appropriately, then labeled each individual eyedrop bottle with an OD and OS. On the medication Kardex, we circled OD in red (keeping OS in black) on all of his orders. Then when we administered the medications, we checked each bottle carefully against the Kardex. We also told Leon the name of the drug just before instilling it, providing a final check as well as patient education.

To budget time, we scheduled both left and right eyedrops for the same visit whenever possible. But by splitting the times that eye care and oral medications were given, we got to spend a few more minutes with Leon, which made him happy.

Leon's eye problems, of course, were the main reason for his hospitalization, but diabetes, hypertension, and kidney failure were more formidable—if less obvious—foes.

One day, a concerned lab technician called back a fasting blood glucose level in excess of 700 mg/

ml. Still, Leon remained asymptomatic. The following day, though, his glucose dropped to just about 500 mg/ml. He spilled sugar into his urine routinely (although his kidney failure made urine testing unreliable), and his finger-stick results ran positive about half the time—all this despite 55 units of Lente insulin each day.

To complicate his endocrine picture even more, Leon was violently allergic to regular insulin. As a precaution, we pasted allergy warnings on his chart face, on an alert strip above his bed, and on a separate red wristband. We also noted the allergy on his patient-care Kardex, nursing care plan, and medication Kardex. Despite those explicit warnings, a new doctor included "coverage with regular insulin" in Leon's postoperative orders. Luckily, the countersigning nurse caught the error and alerted Leon's surgeon. After that experience, we told Leon to make sure the person who administers

"Nothing's more frightening than hearing only footsteps," Leon told us once. So we always made a point of saying "Hello" when we entered his room and "Good bye, Leon" when we left.

his insulin also reports the type and dosage to him before the injection. Whenever possible, the medication nurse would ask a second nurse to compare the medication order to the vial label and dose in the syringe before medicating Leon.

Although he understood the importance of maintaining insulin-glucose balance through proper diet, Leon found eating a chore, especially after his operation. Restricted to a 2-gram sodium, low-fat, low-cholesterol, 1,800 calorie, American Diabetes Association diet—with protein restrictions imminent if kidney failure progressed—Leon

would sadly ask us, "What's left?" when we discussed his food choices. Maybe we couldn't alter the limitations of his prescribed diet, but we could get him dietary consultation. The dietitian interviewed him and listed the foods he preferred within each permissible category. From then on, Leon tolerated his diet with good-natured joking.

As you know, preventing emesis is critical to any vitrectomy patient because of the rising pressure it creates in the eye. To combat nausea, Leon followed a pregnancy morning-sickness diet. He'd start out with a dry food, such as salt-free crackers. Leon usually drank tea with most meals, but occasionally he'd sip a carbonated diet soda in between. He limited the amount of food he consumed at any one time by saving a piece of fresh fruit or some salad for later.

To prevent vomiting, we treated even mild nausea as early and as aggressively as possible. For postanesthesia retching, we gave Leon intramuscular Compazine with good results.

Of course, his obligatory prone posture for 72 hours after the vitrectomy created havoc for Leon's digestion. But he actually found that position more tolerable than the only alternative—sitting up with his head facedown between two pillows on the tray table. After lunch and dinner, Leon's brother massaged his back and legs, which helped relax Leon and, we hoped, soothe his digestion.

We took his temperature, pulse, and respirations at least once per shift, and his blood pressure every 4 hours. Before administering antihypertensive medications, we double-checked the blood pressure readings carefully and withheld one or more medications when his pressure dipped below 140/90. We routinely checked Leon for occipital headache and decreased urine output. The house ophthalmology staff performed a progressive retinopathy check during funduscopic examinations. Also, Leon was frequently checked to make certain that his retina was attached, the BSS remained clear, and no further bleeding occured in the eye that had surgery.

Leon's kidneys had been damaged by his diabetes and hypertension. To monitor his renal state, we tallied his output each shift, compared his BUN and creatinine levels with his admission baselines, and observed him frequently for increased nausea, pruritus, headache, or mental changes.

Although he seemed outwardly optimistic, Leon showed subtle signs of depression. He seldom initiated conversation and remained still and withdrawn for hours. He cried when some visitors left, especially when his mother and sister returned to West Virginia. Crying was an important outlet for Leon, and since we knew it would not harm his eyes, we let him cry as much as he needed. During one emotional outpouring, Leon confessed to feelings of guilt because he couldn't help care for his father, who had recently suffered a myocardial infarction.

We contacted the social worker, who confirmed that Leon's major strength lay in his family's cohesiveness, mutual love, and strong religious faith. Radio and television church services provided some spiritual brotherhood, as did the regular visits of one of his brothers, a Baptist minister.

By discharge, Leon was determined to recover—one day at a time.

The prognosis for Leon's eyesight remains guarded even today. Following surgery, the vision in his right eye was corrected to 20/200 with cataract glasses. Unfortunately, he still remains totally blind in his left eye, and his systemic problems still persist. Of course, the kind of rapidly fulminating kidney and cardiovascular damage that Leon experienced during the last half year carries a grave long-term prognosis. But we had reason to be proud. Despite the stress of two eye surgeries and an extended hospitalization, Leon's diabetes, hypertension, and kidney failure did not accelerate from admission-day baselines. His insulin dosage and blood pressure medication levels still remain at preoperative settings.

Chances are we'll never meet a sweeter person than Leon. But as a patient, his potential for crisis was enormous. And giving him the complex, individualized care he needed called for an enormous effort from all the staff.

First: Make the Patient a Believer

FLORETTE E. CRAMER, RN

One truism in nursing is that for our patients to recover, we have to get them to believe they can. But sometimes we have to get them to believe in *us* first.

Dirk Crain taught me that. When he arrived on the intermediate care unit where I'm a head nurse, he wasn't ready to trust anyone. Considering what he'd been through, that wasn't surprising. Some 9 months before, he'd been stricken with Guillain-Barré (GHEE-*yan* bah-RAY) syndrome.

As you may know, this syndrome is characterized by paralysis, which usually occurs within 2 to 14 days of onset. The body's immune system overreacts to an infection, destroying not only the infection source but also the myelin sheaths covering the motor nerves. Varying degrees of paralysis result, although the sensory nerves are seldom affected.

Because Guillain-Barré syndrome can't be cured, the goal of treatment is to control the symptoms, thus stabilizing vital functions until the body itself stops the demyelination and generates new myelin tissue. This regeneration may take from 2 months to 2 years or more, depending on how much of the body's motor function has been lost.

If the patient survives the initial cardiac and respiratory distress, his prognosis is good. Most patients don't have any residual paralysis. The long-term nursing goal, then, is to help the patient rehabilitate his atrophied muscles and deal with psychological problems.

During the acute stage of his illness, Dirk had become a complete quadriplegic, retaining only the ability to blink his eyes, move his lower jaw, and control his elimination. For 5 months, he'd needed a ventilator to breathe.

When he was transferred to our unit from the neurology unit, his paralysis was still quite severe. He could only rotate his head, lift his arms about 6 inches (15 cm) off the bed, flex the extensor muscles of his thighs slightly, and make facial expressions. Long months of inactivity had limited the range of motion in his shoulders, elbows, hands, and knees. His general muscle tone was poor. His swallowing muscles were also affected, so he'd been receiving his antihypertensive medications and feedings through a nasogastric tube.

Dirk had regained respiratory control but still

had a cuffed tracheostomy tube. He'd signal for suctioning every 15 to 30 minutes, pressing a call light switch with his chin.

Dirk rarely tried to speak. Communicating with him meant interpreting his head and hand movements and facial expressions. He would also nod when someone pointed to letters on an alphabet board.

I met Dirk for the first time when I answered his call light the day he was admitted to the unit. He'd been pressing it almost constantly since he'd arrived, each time for suctioning. This middle-aged, tall, and slightly underweight man kept mouthing the word "suction" over and over. He'd been suctioned only 10 minutes earlier.

Thinking he mostly wanted attention, I decided a set schedule might be in order. When I suggested that he be suctioned every hour, he became furious, demanding suctioning at once. To calm him, I suctioned him, repeating that he probably didn't need it done so often.

Our relationship was off to a bad start—I had underestimated how anxious he really was. Before I'd mentioned any changes, I should have given him more time to get to know us—to know we cared about him and that we'd try to meet not only his suctioning needs but any other needs.

The next day wasn't any better for Dirk because he had to face more changes. With the help of two student nurses and a Hoyer lift, I got him out of bed and into a wheelchair. He shook his head angrily throughout the transfer.

Surprisingly, once in the chair, he motioned that he wanted to be wheeled outdoors. A student nurse took him out on the patio, where he remained for an hour and a half, enjoying every minute. It was the first time he'd been outdoors in 9 months. That, at least, was a positive change.

Another patient with Guillain-Barré syndrome had been transferred to the unit the day before, so I assigned Dirk to his room. I thought that since they had been together on the previous unit, they could support each other. I had to think again, fast. The two seemed determined to find out who could get the most attention from us. Remember the record "Dueling Banjos"? Picture "Dueling Call Lights."

After 2 days, I reassigned Dirk to a room at the other end of the unit. Another change, another

angry reaction. He asked a staff member, "Does that Cramer woman work down here, too? I don't like her."

Actually, Dirk didn't seem to like anyone. Apart from suctioning, he resisted everything we tried to do for him. He didn't want a bath, didn't want his mouth cleaned, didn't want to get out of bed.

He was scheduled for sessions in hydrotherapy, physical therapy, and occupational therapy, but he refused to go. And when his doctor tried to explain why he now should have a cuffless tracheostomy tube, Dirk wouldn't listen. Firmly convinced that he couldn't swallow, he believed the cuff prevented mucus and saliva from flowing into his lungs. The doctor decided, however, to replace the tube despite Dirk's reluctance.

This was one too many changes for Dirk. A sullen look, as cold and final as a closed door, settled over him.

At the end of Dirk's first week, I had to admit that the staff's efforts were getting nowhere. I decided I'd personally take over his nursing care. With all the changes he'd been through, maybe he just needed some consistency. If I could get to know him, gain his confidence, and relieve some of his anxiety, he might let us help him.

How could I get to know him, though, if he wouldn't talk? Or would he? One morning, when several of us were moving him out of bed, I heard him make a sound. After he was settled in a chair, I put my finger over his tube and said, "Why don't you try to talk, Dirk?"

He did: "A pillow, please."

Sure, it was a breathless, short whisper, but at least he had made the effort.

I began spending as many spare minutes as possible talking to Dirk, staying past my shift sometimes. A rapport was tentatively taking shape between us as months of bottled-up speech poured out of him.

And he *did* need someone to talk to. His ex-wife had stopped visiting; his 17-year-old son could come only twice a month. Although his best friend did stop in every week, on many days staff members were his sole social contacts.

Gradually, Dirk started trusting me: He let me shave, shampoo, and groom him more often. Now I had to get that trust to work for him.

On the first day of his scheduled hydrotherapy,

for instance, Dirk said, "I can't go. I have a cold." I didn't insist, but I talked to him about the value of hydrotherapy several times in the next few days. Then I told him, "Let's make Monday your deadline for starting hydrotherapy."

When Monday came, Dirk said, "I can't go. What if I need suctioning?"

I countered, "I'll send a nurse with you to hydrotherapy. She can suction you if you need it." He reluctantly agreed.

As I expected, Dirk didn't need suctioning during the half hour of therapy. From that time on, a physical therapist took him to hydrotherapy. Dirk also went to his occupational therapy sessions—with no problems, suctioning or otherwise.

He still tested me occasionally, though. One morning, he said, "It's too cold to go to hydrotherapy today. It's winter." I reminded him that winter doesn't end until late March, and that it was now early February. He'd miss a lot of hydrotherapy sessions. "I don't care what month it is," he said. "I don't think hydrotherapy is any good. So I'm not going."

"Hydrotherapy can seem slow," I said. "But reeducating your muscles will take time, and hydrotherapy is a very important first step. Besides, as your nurse my job is to help you take advantage of as many chances as possible to get well. And I intend to live up to that responsibility. From now on, you're going to hydrotherapy every day."

Dirk looked at me for a long moment, then said, "Okay."

I think that's when Dirk really began to have faith in me—and to share my belief that he could recover. To bolster that belief, I gave him some of the articles I'd found on Guillain-Barré syndrome. They reiterated that the prognosis was good, given time.

I had another reason for my reading: I was searching for ways to combat his paralysis. What procedure should I use first? How could I best motivate him? I decided to rely on my own nursing instincts in planning his care.

My first step was to be sure he'd eat enough to have the energy he'd need. He wasn't gaining any weight from his tube feedings. According to Dirk's doctor, the nasogastric tube could come out as soon as Dirk could swallow normally. He hadn't tasted food since he was stricken with his disease, and he wouldn't try anything by mouth for fear of choking. I gave him a spoonful of ice cream one day, a small taste of pureed carrots the next. Within a week, he could eat enough food by mouth to justify removing the nasogastric tube.

Next, I convinced Dirk to try breathing with his tracheostomy tube plugged. Without his belief in me, he never would have agreed to even try, since he was understandably anxious about his breathing. A few weeks later, when he admitted he could breathe well with his tube plugged, the tube that had been his lifeline for so long was removed.

Now Dirk was making real progress. He became more relaxed. His blood pressure returned to normal range, so his antihypertensive drugs were discontinued.

The gains in rehabilitating Dirk's atrophied muscles came slower. But whenever he showed he could do something for himself—no matter how much struggle was involved—I'd insist that he continue to do it from then on.

For instance, Dirk needed a great deal of help to sit up. Together, we experimented with different techniques to use the muscles he had to his best advantage. With tremendous effort, he managed to pull himself up to a sitting position in bed one day. From then on, I expected him to sit up by himself. On those rare occasions when he just couldn't make it alone, I did help a little, but he still had to work hard.

One morning, a nursing student who was watching Dirk's laborious attempts moved forward to help. I said, "Wait—he can do it himself." As we stood by his bed, Dirk struggled up...and smiled.

Later that day, Dirk said to me, "I'm not sure anymore whether I'm working hard to accomplish new things for myself or just trying to please you."

Whatever his motivation, he kept reaching new plateaus. In physical therapy, he'd progressed from making only slight movements in the hydro-pool to walking between the parallel bars with braces on his legs. At that point, the physical therapy department was short-staffed, so they stopped doing range-of-motion exercises with his still partially locked joints. This roadblock depressed him.

When I asked Dirk to explain the techniques the therapists used, he brightened visibly. I didn't think they sounded too difficult to do on the unit. So, after some instruction from the physical therapy staff, I spent 15 minutes each morning helping Dirk through the exercises. Within 2 months, his shoulders and elbows were functionally free. By then, the occupational therapy staff had trained him to exercise his hands by himself.

As soon as Dirk mastered a new skill, I'd immediately insist that he go on to the next. When you're really in touch with a patient, you come to know his condition so well you can predict what the next accomplishment should be. And because I thought each step through carefully beforehand, I seldom had to change the direction of his rehabilitation.

This consistency reassured Dirk and helped him maintain his belief in me. He never complained that the expectations were too high because, besides checking over the goals with his doctor and therapists, I always talked them over with him.

My *listening* to Dirk was even more crucial in forming realistic goals. His input let me know whether what I was trying would work. For instance, according to Dirk's physical therapy schedule, he had to practice walking in the afternoon. At one point he became very discouraged, saying, "Even with two therapists to help me and with leg braces on, my legs are weak and wobbly. It's just a waste of time. I'm not getting better at all."

I asked his therapist to walk with Dirk in the morning instead of the afternoon, since he'd probably have more strength and be less tired then. The results were immediate: Dirk could walk between the parallel bars—without braces.

Several days later, I suggested that Dirk lie down in bed after lunch daily, rest for about 2 hours, then try walking again. At first, he complained that it wasn't worth all the trouble of getting in and out of bed, but I asked him to at least give the idea a try. He said, "Okay, if it'll make you happy." In fact, it made both of us happy because he found he was much stronger after his rest and could walk in the afternoons, too. The afternoon rest became an integral part of his therapy.

Dirk's progress settled into a steady, sure rhythm. Sometimes, though, I did have to remind him of where he'd been the month before to keep his spirits up. At first I tried to counter every negative remark with a positive one. Then I learned to listen more patiently, sympathize with some of his frustrations, and encourage him to keep going.

And he did. Nearly 2 years and 9 months after his admission, Dirk was discharged. A week later, he went back to work full time as an engineer at a large aircraft company. The last time he called, he said he's still using a walker and his hands aren't fully functioning, but he drives himself to work every morning. I expect the demands of everyday living will help improve his physical mobility even further. More good news: He's also returned to graduate school, hoping to complete his doctorate in industrial psychology within the next year.

Dirk has almost come full circle after his long bout with Guillain-Barré syndrome. He will, I'm sure, complete the circle. His remarkable progress has made a believer of him. In fact, he now believes in himself as much as he once believed in me—and that's nearly as much as I believe in him.

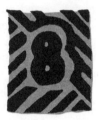

Numidia Looked Like a Model, but She Wasn't a Model Patient

VERONICA HUNKO, RN

In theory, the model patient would be friendly, cooperative, and respond well to treatment. In real life, though, patients can be cranky, uncooperative—and can develop complications that they don't seem even to *want* to recover from. Pretty Numidia Annaba, who wanted to be a fashion model, was anything but a model patient.

A willowy, dark-haired girl in her early twenties, Numidia was admitted from the emergency department one night with a 104° fever of unknown origin. She complained that she'd had a severe headache for several days. Blood cultures were drawn, and a spinal tap done, but there was no elevation in spinal column pressure. After 2 days, Numidia slipped into a coma. Subsequent culture reports led to a diagnosis of tuberculous meningitis.

Numidia's husband was devastated. Every day he sat by her bedside, holding her limp hand and murmuring softly to her in French. He watched us caring for her, and asked about everything we did.

Normally, we ask visitors to leave while we perform nursing procedures, but Mr. Annaba seemed so lost and helpless, we let him stay. We explained the intravenous treatment and the tube feedings, and he, in turn, told us things about his wife that helped later with our care program.

Married only a few years, the Annabas had come to New York City recently from Algeria. He worked as a waiter, and she was a hairdresser. "But her dream was to become a model," Numidia's husband said, pulling some of her modeling photographs from his pocket.

The photographs showed our patient at her loveliest—posing in the park, her large, dark eyes accented with just the right amount of makeup, her stance graceful and confident. We wondered: Would she ever look that way again?

During the 2 weeks Numidia was comatose, we encouraged her husband to keep talking to her. "We don't know for sure that she can't hear you," we told him. We all felt better listening to his quiet murmurings as we administered routine care and did all we could to prevent further complications.

Gradually, Numidia came around. But even when she was fully awake, she wouldn't speak. Her husband talked to her in French, and we carried on lively one-way conversations in English (the Annabas spoke both languages fluently). To give our conversation program continuity, we noted on Numidia's chart what we'd said to her, so each shift could repeat the same sentences. We thought that if she heard the same words over and over, she'd be less confused, and might begin to respond.

One month after she'd awakened from her coma, I greeted her with my usual, "Good morning, Numidia." Out of the blue, she responded, in perfect English, "Good morning, nurse." Excitedly, I called every member of the staff to her bedside. One by one, she greeted them. Although this simple phrase was all Numidia would say, it was the first sign of progress. So we redoubled our efforts to correct her other behavioral problems.

Numidia had regressed to childlike behavior. She refused to use silverware and would eat only with her hands. She'd gladly take a piece of candy, but refused her medicine. She cried when she wanted a drink. She was strong enough to sit in a wheelchair for short periods, if she was supported, but she deliberately slid down in the chair when the staff was busy with other patients. She was incontinent, and played with her feces.

Although we had to keep records of everything that happened to Numidia—both positive and negative—we decided to emphasize the positive. Numidia's appetite was practically nonexistent, and she'd lost 35 pounds during her stay. So, to encourage her to eat, we noted on her chart foods she accepted well. We noted, too, whenever we had success with the bedpan or cooperation with our attempts to sit her up.

She was too weak to be sent for therapy every day, so we asked the therapist to teach us how to exercise her in her room, and we put bilateral splints on her legs to prevent footdrop.

We wanted her to have round-the-clock attention, so on every shift one nurse would exercise her, one nurse would give her bowel training, and one nurse would teach her to feed herself. By having specific assignments, we felt that we gave better, more continuous care.

Numidia's husband was worried about her speech. "Good morning," was still the only English phrase she'd utter, but she'd occasionally babble in French—mostly incoherently, her husband told us.

We asked him to bring in some magazines, and we cut out pictures of familiar things—a house, a dog, a chair, a baby. We also cut out action pictures and simple words—sit, eat, walk—we hoped she'd identify with. Then we put the pictures on the wall, and the nurses on each shift asked

Numidia had regressed to childlike behavior. She refused to use silverware and would eat only with her hands. She'd gladly take a piece of candy, but refused her medicine. She cried when she wanted a drink. She was incontinent, and played with her feces.

Numidia to name them. We praised her lavishly for correct answers (we'd learned the French words for our pictures, so she could answer in either French or English).

But even though Numidia was beginning to take an interest in her surroundings, she still took no interest in her appearance—glaringly abnormal behavior for someone who wanted to be a model. Remembering the modeling photographs, we asked Numidia's husband to bring some of her clothes from home, and we dressed her in them, even though she was still totally incontinent. Mr. Annaba took her soiled daytime clothes home and laundered them himself, and we washed her nightclothes at the hospital.

We shampooed and set her beautiful hair twice a week, and every day we dressed her and put her wheelchair in the center of activity. On quiet days, we'd sit her by the nurses' station while we worked. Like a child, she was captivated by what was going on around her. But she still couldn't sit in a wheelchair without being supported, and became hypotensive if she sat up for more than an hour.

At first, Numidia complained about having her hair washed, but after a few weeks, she began to look forward to it. She smiled coyly when her husband brought her flowers, and we were greatly encouraged when one day she remarked about a nurse's new hairdo.

Our patient had recovered from an upper respiratory infection, urinary tract infection, and gastrointestinal bleeding, and she had no decubiti or contractures. But just when she seemed well on the road to recovery, she developed a fungus infection. A blood culture revealed Candida in her blood stream. Gravely, the doctor told Mr. Annaba that the infection had invaded Numidia's brain, and that she probably had irreversible brain damage. He said that Numidia would need extensive rehabilitation if she were to progress any further,

 But even though Numidia was beginning to take an interest in her surroundings, she still took no interest in her appearance—abnormal behavior for someone who wanted to be a model. Remembering the modeling photographs, we dressed her in clothes from home, even though she was totally incontinent.

and he suggested that she be transferred to a rehabilitation hospital.

We were crushed by the news. After working with Numidia for 6 months, we'd reached an end

point. We hated to see her leave our hospital, but we knew we couldn't do anything else for her.

Numidia's husband fought the idea of a transfer. He'd come to trust us and felt secure with the care we were giving his wife. We could understand his fears, so we suggested he visit the rehabilitation hospital and report back to us. Then we asked our hospital's social worker to contact the rehabilitation hospital and arrange for Numidia's husband to visit her as often as he liked.

When Mr. Annaba filled us in on all the programs the rehabilitation hospital had to offer, he relieved *our* uncertainties. We gave our patient a good-bye party and sent her on her way. The copy of her chart was as thick as a PDR, and the discharge note spelled out all her progress and difficulties, including her special likes and dislikes as well as her therapies.

Numidia had been our patient for 6 months, and we couldn't easily forget her. So about a month after her discharge, another staff nurse and I went to see her.

She was sitting in a wheelchair without restraints, and she smiled pleasantly and said hello to us. But there wasn't a hint of recognition in her eyes—she didn't remember us.

We asked to speak to her doctor, who complimented us on our nurses' notes and praised us for the extra effort we'd shown in caring for Numidia. We told him she didn't seem to remember us. "Could this be because of the brain damage?" we asked. The doctor told us he wasn't convinced Numidia *had* brain damage, but only time would tell.

Then the doctor introduced us to the nursing staff, and we all went through Numidia's chart. We pointed out our triumphs—even the small ones—and explained what we'd done to achieve each success. We also told them about our failures—the biggest one, we thought, was the bowel training program. Numidia was totally incontinent when she left our hospital, and she still was, 1 month later.

The nurses told us they were following the same bowel training program we'd used—taking Numidia to the bathroom at the same times every day—but with no success. We told them about Numidia's dream of becoming a model, and about how well-groomed she'd been before her illness. We suggested that they dress her in her own clothes, as we'd done. They were anxious to try our idea, and we all hoped that wearing her own clothes might give Numidia the incentive to become continent.

The nurses urged us to come again—no one but Mr. Annaba ever visited, they said. We returned several times, and each visit brought an improved picture of our patient. The doctor at our hospital had been wrong—Numidia obviously didn't have brain damage.

Numidia had gained strength and was beginning to stand alone. She'd learned to dress herself (she was wearing her own clothes now), and the nurses said she combed her hair every morning before getting out of bed. Her appetite improved, and she was able to wheel herself to the cafeteria. In fact, she gained so much weight the nurses had to make her cut down on sweets. But, most important, she was no longer incontinent.

Eventually, Numidia looked forward to our visits—even though she still didn't remember we'd been her nurses. When she knew we were coming, she'd put on her makeup. By our fourth visit, she was talking as though we were dear friends. She showed us pictures of her family and spoke about going home.

Mr. Annaba told us that Numidia remembered

nothing of what had happened to her, but that her mental status had greatly improved. She had some residual effects from the illness—a partial hearing loss, diminished vision, and a slight limp—but after she learned to walk with a cane, she was allowed to go home for weekends in preparation for her discharge.

One week after she'd left the rehabilitation hospital, Numidia and her husband came to visit us. We could hardly believe that the smartly dressed, sparkling young woman was the helpless, whining child we'd cared for 1½ years before.

The Annabas had come to say good-bye—they were returning to Algeria to visit their families. And they wanted to thank us one last time.

"I know I owe you a great deal," Numidia told us. "And I only wish I could remember how good you were to me. But I can't remember anything about the 6 months I was in the hospital."

We remembered, though. True, some of our memories of caring for our less-than-model patient were painful ones. But, as Numidia walked away from us looking like the girl in the modeling photographs, how good it felt to know that our patience and perseverance had helped her look that way again.

Mrs. Hixon Was More than "The CVA in 251"

SUE COLLIER, RN, BSN

Most of us, at sometime, have used a kind of verbal shorthand to identify a patient—"the CVA in 251" or "the M.I. in 330."

I guess I never realized how depersonalizing this is until the day Mrs. Hixon was admitted to our critical care unit with a stroke. I would never have thought of calling Mrs. Hixon "the CVA in 251" because I *knew* Mrs. Hixon. I knew the whole family. Her husband was a florist and Mrs. Hixon worked in the shop with him. She had a daughter about to be married; a son in college. Then, too, I shared those first painful hours with the family. I saw the agony and disbelief on their faces as they walked into her room and saw the person so dear to them lying there, desperately sick and helpless. For me, Mrs. Hixon was not a "CVA," but a very real person who happened to be our patient.

For many days, Mrs. Hixon's condition remained critical. Finally, when we were sure she would live, the question then became: what would the quality of that life be? Here was a 46-year-old woman, paralyzed on her right side, and with severe expressive aphasia.

One nursing care plan now called for heavy emphasis on retraining the patient to do as much for herself as possible. This was more of a task than any of us anticipated. Mrs. Hixon seemed determined to ignore the nursing staff. She tolerated the daily hospital routine only because she had no other choice. If ever we tried to get her to work with us, her one reply was an emphatic "No, no, no!" We understood that this repeated response could just be a form of automatic speech, which frequently occurs in aphasia. Frankly, however, we suspected it summed up the patient's deepest emotional response to her plight.

We held a number of conferences about this problem and decided the first thing to do was provide continuity of care on all three shifts. We hoped that as Mrs. Hixon came to recognize us and realize she could rely on us, her confidence in herself—and us—would be regenerated. We also felt that by using the same staff, we'd have a better chance of recognizing the patient's unspoken nursing needs. Two other things we agreed on. The first was that we would carefully explain to Mrs. Hixon everything we were going to do and how she could help us. We felt it was important for her to understand that we weren't just doing things *to* her—but *with* her. The second thing we determined was how we would speak to her. When a patient is aphasic, it's all too easy to slip into the feeling that she is also deaf and possibly mentally retarded. This is not true and, although we made a point of speaking clearly and in short sentences, we still spoke to her as adult-to-adult, and in a normal tone of voice.

As the weeks passed and Mrs. Hixon became stronger, our plan for continuity of care seemed to be working. We felt she now recognized us individually and she began smiling when we did something that pleased her. We were encouraged and felt we had gained her trust—the first step toward gaining her cooperation.

About a month after her admission, I served Mrs. Hixon her first tray of food. It was only soup and Jello, but her face beamed at this step back toward normal living. Her happiness was to be short-lived, however, and I saw anguish fill her eyes as she silently commanded her right hand to pick up the spoon. But the hand just lay there, still and lifeless. In working with Mrs. Hixon, we had often explained to her that she'd had a stroke, but she had been using denial as her way of coping. Now, with the arm put to the test, she could no longer deny the truth. We had the job of helping her accept the reality of her situation.

Again, I explained to her that her right side was weakened from her stroke, but that she could feed herself with her left hand for the time being. Reluctantly, *most* reluctantly, she raised the soup spoon to her lips only to find that the soup ran out the right side of her mouth and down the front of her new nightgown. Quickly, I collected several more napkins and a narrow-tipped teaspoon. I spread the napkins, stacking them one on top of another until they looked like one napkin with the thickness of ten. I placed my "supernapkin" across the front of her gown and secured it with two small safety pins. I wanted to avoid anything that she could possibly construe as a bib. Mrs. Hixon's self-image, I felt, had been battered enough. Next, I showed her how to use the smaller teaspoon, directing the tip of it into the left side of her mouth where she had more feeling and greater muscular control. This eliminated about three quarters of the annoying dribbling. I made a notation on her

care plan to use the "supernapkin" and the narrow-tipped spoon. I also directed that all silverware and beverages be placed on the left side of her tray for easier accessibility.

As Mrs. Hixon's condition continued to improve, she began physical, occupational and speech therapy. I sometimes sat in on the classes to see what lessons might be reinforced on the unit. In a way, it was like teaching a child how to walk, talk, dress and care for herself. She did have some use of her right leg, so we began retraining her to walk, using a tripod cane. Because the patient's sense of gravity had been altered, her balance was precarious, and we had to protect her from falling. At first, two of us tried supporting her as she walked but this proved too awkward. We then strapped a wide belt around her waist and stationed one person on each side to hold onto the belt. This made movement much easier but still provided the patient with

 I served Mrs. Hixon her first tray of food, and her face beamed at this step back toward normal living. Her happiness was short-lived, however. When she silently commanded her right hand to pick up the spoon, the hand just lay there, still and lifeless.

some degree of stability and sense of security. Gradually, as Mrs. Hixon gained self-confidence and her coordination inproved, we dispensed with the belt and later, with the "escort service."

When Mrs. Hixon was relearning how to redress herself, it initially took her an hour. With much practice and with guidance from the occupational therapist, this time finally dropped to 25 minutes.

Even so, I confess I practically had to sit on my hands as I watched her struggle, one-handed, with her pants and the buttons on her blouse. It would have been so much faster to do it for her, but she had to learn, and I had to let her. The occupational therapist made a helpful suggestion—all-elastic brassieres, available in most large department stores. Mrs. Hixon was delighted at how easily they slipped on, and even more pleased that she could do it all by herself!

Because her speech problem seemed to be the most frustrating to her, we concentrated on it hardest. A speech therapist worked with her for 1 hour daily and, though the sessions were invaluable, a stroke patient's readiness for learning is not something that can always be scheduled at a specific time. Mrs. Hixon's attention span was short and tended to be sporadic. We realized that the staff and the family would have to serve as reinforcement for every lesson if Mrs. Hixon were to progress.

We asked Mr. Hixon to bring in familiar snapshots from home. He brought in pictures of the Hixon house and car and each member of the family—down to and including the beloved family

 I suddenly realized that her joking was a way of covering up her feelings of inadequacy and fear she would not be able to say what she wanted—not now—or ever. The harder she tried, the more upset and anxious she became.

pooch, Rodger. We identified each picture on the back in large letters, fashioning the first of many sets of flash cards. To use the cards, we would first show Mrs. Hixon the picture, then have her watch our mouth as we slowly pronounced the word on the back. She would repeat the word once with us, and once by herself while reading it from the back of the flash card. Often, we would find her alone just looking at the pictures and trying to pronounce the words all by herself. Not only did this help her pass many long hours but she was learning all the while.

I realized how little I knew about aphasia and, in reading up on the subject, came across much useful information to share with the staff and family. I learned that although we can't make blanket generalizations (each care plan must take into consideration the individual's personality, degree of impairment, and so on), there are some standard approaches aphasics seem to respond well to. For example, aphasics do better with people they're familiar with, and on a one-to-one basis. They can profit from the repetition of a statement if it doesn't occur too quickly. We must give the first statement a good chance to sink in before repeating it a second or third time. Because aphasics are less able to block out other happenings in the environment, we should try to minimize extraneous noise—turn off the radio or TV, shut the door to the corridor—before trying to talk to them. Aphasics also profit from our use of body language. When we would tell Mrs. Hixon we were taking her down the hall for physical therapy, for example, we would also point down the hall to give her a second chance to grasp our meaning.

We incorporated these and other points into our care plan; still it could be very discouraging. Mrs. Hixon's favorite phrase when she didn't know the answer was "let's see," followed by a cute little laugh. This became her pat answer for almost everything, and I soon became exasperated with her for seeming to joke all the while I was trying to be serious and help her. One day I spoke to her about this, and she began to cry. I felt terrible because I suddenly realized that her joking was a way of covering up her feelings of inadequacy and fear she would not be able to say what she wanted—not now—or ever. This realization made me all the more determined to help Mrs. Hixon in every way I could. Yes, I *was* working very hard but surely the great struggle was hers.

Try as she might, however, there were many times when she was just not able to tell us what it was she wanted. The harder she tried, the more upset and anxious she became. Just telling her "that's all right—you'll think of it later" was no solution as far as she was concerned. It only made her more tense and frustrated. To deal with this problem, we developed a game of sorts. More often than not, the "mystery word" turned out to be something she wanted. We began by asking her "If you had it, what would you do with it?" Mrs. Hixon would then reply with a gesture such as pretending to be eating, combing her hair, and so on. We, in turn, would make guesses. This system wasn't foolproof by any means. It took a lot of time, but it helped channel her frustrations in a positive manner and give her the feeling that we really did care about her needs and wants. Patience on the part of the patient, as well as of the nurse, has definitely got to be the prime ingredient in the care of an aphasic.

As Mrs. Hixon progressed, we watched with mixed feelings, knowing that each step brought her closer to one more difficult hurdle: depression. Once a patient has recovered enough to fully comprehend the extent of her illness, she is often overwhelmed by the change in her life. Mrs. Hixon was no exception. There were days when she would cry quietly, and there were days when she would keep asking, "Why did this have to happen?"

knowing there was really no answer. With any loss, it's important for the individual to pass through a process of grieving. As nurses, we must recognize this need and be supportive when it occurs. We had no pat answers for Mrs. Hixon. All we could do was acknowledge her feelings and be honest with her. Sometimes, just sitting quietly holding her hand seemed to help.

Looking back now, I marvel at Mrs. Hixon's courage and perseverance. Nothing was easy for her; yet, she kept trying. As the weeks passed slowly into months, she continued her progress and we were all very proud of her.

Certainly we'd taught her a lot, but she taught us much, too. From her, I learned the incredible frustration, suffering and loneliness the aphasic stroke patient experiences and the seemingly insurmountable obstacles she must face in overcoming her handicap.

After working with Mrs. Hixon, I don't think I'll ever be able to think of another person as just the "M.I. in 330" or the "CVA in 251." I think I now really appreciate that each patient is a very special person whose care must be highly individualized. Because of Mrs. Hixon, I think I am a better nurse and a more understanding human being. She is one patient I'm not likely to forget. She's my mother.

Andy Was a Fighter – in More Ways than One

MARIBELLE LEAVITT, RN, MS

Severely burned patients are always critically ill. The never-ending schedule of burn treatments can wear out even the bravest patient, the strongest nurse. And seeing a patient in constant pain is painful for the nurse, too. Caring for Andy was exhausting and painful for both of us.

Fifteen-year-old Andy came to our burn unit after a freak accident. Somehow, he'd fallen into a partly filled bathtub and had been knocked unconscious. When his mother found him, he was still unconscious, lying on his right side in 2 inches of scalding water. Andy had second- and third-degree burns over the entire right side of his body.

We placed Andy in a private room, in reverse isolation. At first, we were all impressed with his courage and strength. Although the dressing changes and tub baths must've been excruciating for him, he never complained.

We'd carefully remove his dressings three times a day, almost feeling his pain, and we'd watch his eyes fill with tears and his muscles tighten. Then we'd carefully lower him into a tub filled with saline solution and antibacterial cleanser and *our* eyes would fill with tears, knowing how agonizing the salt solution felt on his raw, burned skin.

But after 2 weeks, Andy's courage began to dwindle. The exhausting routine of painful dressing changes and tub baths became unbearable for him. Instead of silently enduring the treatments, he started howling as soon as we approached his bed. And instead of fighting back his tears, he started fighting *us,* pulling away when we tried to change his dressings, screaming when we lowered him into the tub.

Inflicting more pain on Andy—even though the pain was unavoidable—made us feel like villains. I'm sure I wasn't the only nurse who groaned inwardly, and then felt guilty, when she was assigned to Andy.

Although we had a detailed physical care plan for Andy, as for all our patients, we hadn't yet worked out a strategy for dealing with his problem behavior. Whenever an emotional crisis arose or a patient's behavior became difficult, we responded on the spot, using our ingenuity.

Andy's biggest crisis came after he'd been on the unit 2 weeks. I was removing his dressings one day, paying particular attention to the most severely burned area—his external ear. The skin looked gray and sticky, and dead tissue kept sloughing off. With a sick feeling, I suspected the ear wasn't healing; that it might be dead. The doctor confirmed my fears—Andy would lose his ear. What a blow this would be to a teenager's self-image. Now we had to mobilize our problem-solving efforts to help Andy face probably the biggest crisis in his life.

Helping a brave and uncomplaining Andy through this crisis would've been hard enough. But now we had a new Andy to deal with. How could we tell a weary, regressed teenager that his ear was, literally, about to fall off?

At this point in his care, I'd spent more time with Andy than any of the other nurses. He seemed to relate well to me—probably because I was one of the youngest nurses on the unit. But Andy needed more than a nurse, he needed a friend. He'd been transferred from a small hospital miles away, so his widowed mother and younger sister visited only once a week. Because he was so far from home, his classmates rarely visited, and we had no other teenage patients on the unit. Andy had some important adolescent needs going unmet, so we had to be mother, father, and friend to him.

Before we could tell Andy about losing his ear, we first had to calm him down during dressing changes. I decided to try "anticipatory guidance"—telling him exactly what I was going to do, down to the minutest detail—so he could prepare himself for the next step in his treatment and for the pain. Then I thought I'd try to "talk him through" his dressing changes, like an obstetrical nurse talks her patients through labor and delivery. Of course, as soon as I walked into Andy's room with the dressing cart, he let out a howl like a trapped animal.

"I know this hurts," I said soothingly. "But we have to change your dressings for you to get better." He stopped howling, but his eyes were panicky. I told him I'd explain everything I was doing, and that, with his help, I felt sure we could get through the ordeal quickly.

Andy cried softly, and as I tried to remove the first set of bandages, he cringed and jumped away. Then I had another idea. Maybe the deep breathing techniques used in natural childbirth would help

him. Concentrating on breathing would take his mind off the pain, and also give him some control over the situation. So I gave Andy a crash course, telling him to focus on an object in the room, and then inhale and exhale rhythmically. He caught on quickly.

"Now you know how to breathe just like an expectant mother," I told him. He actually managed a weak smile.

I began removing his dressings again, slowly, while we *both* breathed deeply. When a bandage was stuck, I'd say, "Hang on, Andy, this one's a toughie," or "This will take about 10 more seconds, why don't you count them out." I talked and we breathed for 1½ hours while I removed the bandages, soaked him in the tub, and reapplied the dressings. We were both exhausted, but not nearly as tired as the day before, when Andy was still fighting.

I couldn't believe my idea had worked so well. The breathing had calmed *me,* too. As I left his room, Andy said, "I don't want anybody but you changing my dressings." I'll admit, I felt pleased.

But even though I was pleased and proud my plan had worked, I had an uneasy feeling it'd worked almost *too* well, because Andy started telling everyone that I'd discovered a "miracle" cure for pain, and that I was the only nurse who could perform this miracle.

We'd begun bending the rules a bit to give Andy a chance to socialize. After his baths and dressing changes, I'd wrap him in sterile sheets and wheel him into the hall by the nurses' station. Whenever another patient or a staff member passed by, he'd tell them about the breathing and what a miracle it was.

Naturally, the other nurses wanted to know the details, and I'd planned to tell them, but in far less glowing terms than Andy's. So, Andy and I demonstrated our deep breathing, and the other nurses gave it a try. At this point, if I'd told them that reciting the Gettysburg Address during dressing changes made Andy cooperate, I think they'd have gladly complied.

Although Andy still insisted I was his "special" nurse, I explained that I couldn't stay with him night and day—that other nurses would have to change his dressings, too. He looked hurt and panicky again, but finally agreed to let the other nurses change his dressings, if they promised to breathe with him.

Andy was acting like himself again—talking and joking with the staff, visiting with the other patients. But the other male patients were years older, and the only people near his age were the nurses. We knew he needed a young man to talk to, a sort of surrogate brother. So we asked Dr. Hamlin, one of the younger residents, if he'd be Andy's "anchor" doctor.

Dr. Hamlin's relationship with Andy was like a coach's relationship with a player. When the doctor debrided Andy's burns—the procedure Andy feared most—the doctor would say, "Come on kid, you can do it." And Andy did. While we mothered Andy, the doctor coached him; and the combination worked.

Now that Andy was himself again, we had to deal with the problem of his ear. Bluntly saying, "You're going to lose your ear any day," was, of course, out of the question. So we broke the news to him little by little.

We'd remove the dressings from his ear and say, "The external ear doesn't look good, Andy." We always emphasized *external* so he'd know he wasn't losing every part of his ear. At first, he was noncommittal, and we worried that maybe he didn't understand, or worse, didn't *want* to understand. I even showed him his ear in a mirror, but he didn't seem shocked, or even interested, and never asked to see it again.

Then he began asking questions. "How does the ear look today?" he'd ask hopefully. And we'd answer truthfully, "It doesn't seem to be healing." Finally, we told him his external ear was dead, that we were sure he'd lose it, and finally, Andy cried. For the next few days he cried every time we mentioned his ear, but we felt he'd made the first step toward accepting the terrible news.

I was with Andy the day his ear came off. As I helped him into the tub, he lightly brushed the right side of his head with his hand and his external ear fell into the water. I quickly scooped it up and wrapped it in gauze. "Your ear just fell off, Andy,"

I said. "Really?" he replied, obviously not stricken. After his bath, I took the ear and quickly disposed of it. Andy hadn't even asked to see it.

Andy was now ambulatory, and as we walked from the tub room past the nurses' station, he calmly told the nurses, "Well, the ear finally fell off today." Even though we'd been prepared for weeks, his matter-of-fact announcement left us a bit speechless.

Shortly before his discharge, Andy became quite modest, and we respected his modesty, knowing it was a sign he was regaining a healthy self-image. For 6 weeks, coping with almost constant pain had been Andy's main concern, and being dressed in only bandages and being bathed by young female nurses hadn't mattered to him. But now that he wasn't in constant pain, he acted like most 15-year-olds—asking for a robe, saying "excuse me" when he undressed in front of us.

He continued to progress well. Most of his skin grafts "took," and he began looking willingly in the mirror for the first time since his admission. The right side of his body was badly scarred, but he seemed to accept this. His face had been burned only as far as the hairline—from the end of his eyebrow to his jawline—so he was still a handsome boy.

We explained that the hair on the right side of his head wouldn't grow back, but he didn't seem to mind the idea of wearing a hairpiece. We also told him that after his skin healed, he'd get a prosthetic ear, and later, if he wanted, he could have an artificial ear constructed. Andy decided that he wanted to return in 6 months for ear reconstruction surgery.

After 1½ months on our unit, Andy was discharged. Although I never saw him again, his memory stays with me. For me, every burn patient is Andy—vulnerable, dependent, walking a line between control and regression, hope and despair.

Nurses sometimes walk that line too, except we *have* to be strong when our patients' courage falters. Andy taught me as much about strength and courage as I taught him—maybe more.

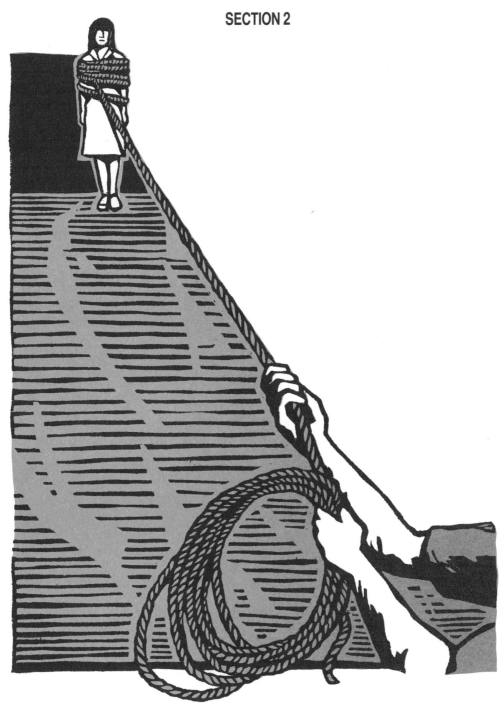

EMOTIONALLY DEMANDING PATIENTS

Our Affection for Mrs. Johns Was Hindering Our Nursing Care

JUDITH EFFKEN, RN

Surely we've all been suitably impressed with the importance of the nurse's attitude toward the patient—how it can directly affect her recovery.

But the nurse-patient relationship is a two-way street. What of the patient's attitude toward *herself* and how *that* can affect the spirit of a whole nursing team? This is what we saw at work in our relationship with Mrs. Johns.

Over a 4-year period, Mrs. Johns had been a frequent patient in our acute-care unit. On her first stay with us, she had a pacemaker inserted for arteriosclerotic heart disease with heart block. At another time, she was admitted with a myocardial infarction. Later, when arteriograms showed total occlusion of her superficial femoral and left internal iliac arteries, she'd been given an axillo-femoral graft. This artificial graft ran from the left axillary artery to the right femoral artery. It could be felt as a tube, 1 inch in diameter, along the left side of her chest and abdomen, crossing the pelvis.

She also had had a left popliteal bypass graft in which the saphenous vein was used to connect the left femoral artery and the popliteal at the ankle level. Several times when the bypass became obstructed, Mrs. Johns returned for embolectomies, and finally a sympathectomy.

During these hospitalizations, we'd come to know—and like—this friendly 63-year-old woman. We knew, for example, that Mrs. Johns and her semi-invalid husband had a warm relationship. Although they were estranged from their only child, the Johns all but worshipped their grandchildren. Mrs. Johns was never without her grandmother's bracelet, whose dangle charms showed the name and birthdate of each grandchild. Always cooperative and cheerful, Mrs. Johns was interested in all the floor activities and was personally interested in each member of the staff. After her husband and her grandchildren, Mrs. Johns' two compelling pleasures were card-playing and smoking. She'd play solitaire until visiting hours, then she and Mr. Johns played gin. Against all doctor's orders, she continued to smoke. As she ruefully explained, she "was hooked."

After Mrs. Johns' last embolectomy, a visiting nurse had been assigned to the Johns. It was she who notified the doctor when she discovered a profuse, purulent discharge draining from Mrs. Johns' groin graft site.

We knew that Mrs. Johns was a chronically sick woman; and from the visiting nurse's report, we knew that the Johns did not follow a good nutritional diet. Still, we were taken aback at the change in her. Normally a slender little person, Mrs. Johns now appeared emaciated. Ordinarily friendly and alert, she was now listless and passive. For the first time, she wasn't wearing her grandmother's bracelet.

A culture of her infected groin area showed *Staphylococcus aureus* coagulation positive, so our first job was to try to clear up the infection. Observing strict wound isolation, we conducted antibiotic therapy and local irrigations.

During our procedures, Mrs. Johns was withdrawn. She dozed and slept most of the day, her hands restlessly picking at the covers. The minute she awakened, she asked for pain medication which promptly put her to sleep again. She hardly ate. The dietician came in every day to suggest different foods that might tempt Mrs. Johns, but she seemed unable to even participate in that simple decision. No matter what we brought her, the trays returned almost untouched.

After a week, the surgeon became concerned about Mrs. Johns' dependence on the codeine she was getting. Since she could no longer pinpoint or describe her pain, we suspected that she was experiencing less discomfort now and was using the analgesic to retreat from the anxiety and depression she felt. The surgeon switched her to Talwin.

Still, Mrs. Johns dozed and was unresponsive. We asked Mr. Johns to bring in her grandmother's bracelet. She barely acknowledged it. He tried to get her to play cards but she nodded off almost before the hand was dealt. "Can't you *do* something," he asked. We all felt so helpless.

Mrs. Johns' bypass remained obstructed but, because the past embolectomies had not worked, the surgeons did not think another advisable. The initial coolness and slight discoloration of the left foot worsened until one morning an actual line of demarcation could be seen. The doctors then decided that amputation was necessary. Three and a half weeks after Mrs. Johns was admitted, her left leg was amputated below the knee. The doctors hoped to preserve the rest of the leg and knee joint

for easier rehabilitation.

Within a week, we could see that the stump was not healing well. But we continued to carry out an elaborate irrigation of the stump several times a day. We felt sure Mrs. Johns recognized these as desperation measures. Our physiotherapist had begun Mrs. Johns on exercises of the stump and of the unimpaired leg while lying down, plus bed to chair transfer. Soon Mrs. Johns complained that she was too sleepy or in too much pain to continue. Finally she just refused to open her eyes when the therapist came.

If the physiotherapist felt frustrated, you can imagine how we felt. We were getting nowhere with the groin infection, and the stump was obviously worsening. Mrs. Johns now required complete care for her personal hygiene and even help with eating.

Perhaps of all her care, our failure to get her to eat was the most discouraging. Originally, we encouraged her with comments like "That soup smells so good!" or "Try the roast beef... it's really tender." We also tried the "Would you like a sandwich instead?" route. We pleaded openly, "Please eat, Mrs. Johns. You really must try to eat." We even bribed: "If you'll just finish the soup, then you can rest awhile."

Our approaches were as varied as the members of the nursing team themselves. The only thing unchanging was Mrs. Johns' refusal to eat. She complained that eating only nauseated her. We tried splitting her three meals into six, hoping that smaller portions would not overwhelm her failing appetite. We split her breakfast, for example, into warm cereal and juice at 8 a.m. and poached egg and toast at 10; her lunch into a bowl of soup at 12 noon; ice cream and cookies at 2 p.m.; and so on. Finally we started her on a regimen of high-caloric, high-protein drinks, even substituting them for water when we gave her her pills. All of this had little effect. "Later" was her constant response to our pleas, but it was a "later" that never became "now."

We began to suspect that our affection and sympathy for Mrs. Johns might be keeping us from making appropriate nursing decisions. She could, in her own way, manipulate us. She knew, for example, that once she complained of nausea, we wouldn't try to force her to eat more. She knew that if she complained of pain, we wouldn't withhold her medication. Most of all, she knew how much we respected the healing worth of a patient's sleep and that we hated to wake someone unless necessary. This last ploy she used continually and effectively to block out us... and her chances for recovery. Mrs. Johns was convinced she couldn't make it. Her attitude was beginning to wear off on us.

Everyone was depressed. We had conferences, scheduled and unscheduled, when we'd go over Mrs. Johns' care plan and try to get some new direction... something that would work. One nurse complained that she just couldn't accomplish anything more with Mrs. Johns. Another confided that just seeing Mrs. Johns as she was now made her fight back tears. Another confessed to putting Mrs. Johns' care last among her assigned tasks. These nurses spoke for us all.

Besides her psychological regression, Mrs. Johns now became mentally confused. She heard people talking to her from outside the window. She tried to get out of bed. Finally, she did fall. Although she wasn't hurt, we had no choice but to use a Posey restraint. We'd tried to avoid this last insult to her independence as a person, but now safety demanded it.

We tried to explain our reasoning to Mrs. Johns, but she closed her eyes and turned her face away as if we'd betrayed her. In desperation, we even considered transferring Mrs. Johns to another unit, hoping that another group of nurses might be more effective. We talked this possibility over with Mrs. Johns' physician but concluded that she might interpret this move as rejection and be totally crushed.

We finally ran up the classic white flag of surrender in the face of a frustrating patient: we appended Mrs. Johns' Kardex to read, "Please do not assign to any nurse more than 1 day at a time."

I wish this had brought us some peace of mind, but it didn't. The fact remained that with Mrs. Johns' worsening, our failure faced us every day. In a desperation move, we expanded our next patient conference on Mrs. Johns to include the hospital social worker who knew the Johns, our med-surg clinical specialist, and our patient-education coordinator. We laid out all our feelings: discouragement, inadequacy, and being manipulated

by the patient. We welcomed any suggestions.

Our patient-education coordinator told us of some of her experiences in using a form of behavior modification, based on positive reinforcement. In this program, as you may know, there is no element of punishment. Desirable behavior is immediately rewarded while undesirable behavior is totally ignored.

The coordinator told us we must decide what behavior we seek from the patient, a way to measure that behavior, and an appropriate reward when the patient performs in the desired manner. Almost before she finished, we could feel a change in our attitude.

We knew *exactly* what behavior we wanted. Mrs. Johns could never recover without improving her nutritional status, so our first goal was to get her to eat. Our second goal was to get her reinterested in living. We thought if we could get her to participate in her daily care—if only to wash her face and hands—it would be a good start.

We then discussed how we could measure this behavior and what would be suitable rewards. At the end of the session, we had a new feeling of hope—and this change in Mrs. Johns' care plan:
Goal 1: To increase nutrition.
Approach 1: Give high-caloric feeding to Mrs. J.; if she drinks without assistance, reward with conversation, praise and cigarette if desired. If she does not hold glass and drink, feed it to her without verbal or non-verbal criticism.
Goal 2: To increase self care.
Approach 2: Set up basin for her to wash face and hands; instruct her, then leave room. If she does wash, reward with conversation, praise and cigarette if desired. If she does not wash, remove basin and wash all of body except face and hands. Make no negative comment.

I'd just like to add something about our reward plan. We don't encourage anyone's smoking—especially someone in Mrs. Johns' condition where the vasoconstriction produced by smoking poses a real threat. As Mrs. Johns' physician said when we told him about our plan, however, "Try it. With her status as it is now, we've got very little to lose."

The next morning, Mrs. Green, who was assigned to Mrs. Johns that day, set a basin of water in front of her with the instructions that she should now wash her face and hands before breakfast. Mrs. Green then left the room, saying she'd be back in a few minutes to complete the bath. When Mrs. Green returned, the basin had not been touched, and Mrs. Johns appeared to be dozing. There were no words of reproach. Mrs. Green simply bathed Mrs. Johns—but omitted her face and hands.

The next day, when presented with a basin of water and similar instructions, Mrs. Johns washed her own face and hands and found that Mrs. Green offered her a cigarette and sat down to visit with her. Mrs. Green noted that although the conversation was mostly on *her* part, Mrs. Johns had contributed a few monosyllables. More important, she had participated in her own care. We discussed the care plan in detail at each change-of-shift report to be sure we maintained a consistent approach over the entire 24-hour period.

Within 48 hours, we could measure improvement in Mrs. Johns' dietary intake. We had been offering the high-caloric drink eight times a day, and Mrs. Johns had been taking between 300 and 700 calories. By the end of the second day of our new program, she had taken 1000 calories and was beginning to reach for the glass herself. Six days later, she was regularly holding the glass and was taking 1800 calories a day.

Without being prompted, she now washed her face, hands, *arms and chest*. She asked to do her own denture care. We couldn't help speculating on Mrs. Johns' remarkable—and swift—improvements. We finally concluded that, hazy as Mrs. Johns had been, she'd received the unspoken message of our behavior modification program: "You may have given up on yourself, but we haven't. We still expect things of you because *you can do them*."

In view of Mrs. Johns' returning strength, the surgeon decided to remove the infected bypass graft through the groin. This was successful and ended the drainage. The wound culture turned negative and the area began to granulate.

Mrs. Johns continued to advance psychologically, too. She now asked for her brush and make-up kit. She used cologne. Once more, she seemed to care about how she looked.

The surgeons now scheduled her for an above-knee amputation. We were apprehensive. Would this new blow destroy all we had worked for?

But again Mrs. Johns held on to her gains. We discussed the probable reasons. First, of course, Mrs. Johns now had renewed physical strength because of better nutrition. Then, amputation was no longer a new and shattering experience for her. She realized that she was still the same person— even without part of a leg. And finally, she now knew we counted on *her* to work with us to restore her to health.

We felt the time had come to wean Mrs. Johns away from the high-caloric drink and back to solid food. We discussed this with her. At first she was anxious, fearing that the solid foods would nauseate her again. But we promised to let her go at her own pace. She decided to forego the 8, 12 and 4 drink feedings and try to substitute the regular menu at those times. It was a long time before she could eat an entire meal but, beginning with a few bites, she gradually raised her solid intake. The day she asked for a menu and ordered her own meals was a great day on the unit.

With the stump healing well, the physiotherapist returned for therapy sessions. Mrs. Johns quickly progressed to using a walkerette with help. Finally, she was scheduled for discharge to an extended care facility where it was hoped she could be fitted for a prosthesis.

Nine weeks after Mrs. Johns' admission, we held a farewell party for her. We scheduled the party at 3 p.m. so two shifts could be present. We invited the social worker, physiotherapist, clinical specialist, patient-education coordinator, and Mr. Johns. We had cake, punch and a huge banner reading "good luck, Mrs. J."

As we watched the smiling, well-groomed patient in the wheelchair cut and serve the cake to the guests, we felt proud that our program of positive reinforcement had paid off for Mrs. Johns.

And proud—relieved—that it had paid off for us, too. Because it was only through this program that we were able once again to function effectively as nurses on this most difficult case.

Johnny Is My Most Difficult... and Dearest...Patient

KAREN JEAN BLOOMFIELD, RN

Two-year-old John is my most difficult—and dearest—patient. He's my son. And last year, he was diagnosed as having acute lymphoblastic leukemia. Naturally, you'd understand why John is so dear to me, but I'd like to explain why some aspects of his care are so difficult.

Ever since we learned of John's diagnosis, my husband, who's a doctor, and I have studied all we can about leukemic children. We've found some very good information on how to work with those who are old enough to talk and tell us something of their thoughts and feelings. There seems to be very little literature, however, on the toddler who cannot yet distinguish the external world from himself and who is just breaching the verbalization stage. How can you hope to make one so young understand some of the puzzling things that are happening to him? How can you reassure him when he faces terrifying equipment and strange surroundings? How can you preserve his trust through repeated painful procedures? Through everyday living in this uncharted situation, I've worked out some solutions to some of these problems and I'd like to share them with you.

Let's start with the most obvious difficulty: getting a 2-year-old to take daily oral medications. John's principal drugs, Prednisone, Methotrexate and 6-mercaptopurine, do not come in elixir form for children. And, they're very bitter—especially Prednisone. No amount of crushing, diluting or mixing with ice cream or Jello will disguise the flavor. (We know; we sampled a very tiny amount and immediately understood why John hollered and spat them out.) These vital medications must be taken for years, however, and in view of the daily torment it caused John, the situation was critical.

I decided to try empty gelatin capsules. After experimenting, I found that two whole Prednisone tablets could be dropped easily into one size 0 capsule. The methotrexate tablet is similar in size to the Prednisone but the 6-mercaptopurine tablet is larger. By cutting it in half, however, it, too, fit easily into a gelatin capsule. Even a 2-year-old can swallow the small bullous of a capsule if given enough encouragement.

We explained to John that we knew how awful the pills tasted but that by taking them the new way, there would be no taste. Once he realized that there *was* no taste to the "new" medicine and that I wasn't trying to trick him by sneaking the bad-tasting stuff into his food, he not only took his medicine readily, but began eating better, too.

As a result of this discovery, we try to give all additional medications (if obtainable in correct dosage) via capsule form. The relief of not having to taste the drugs is a great motivation for John. Now we have a "pill time" every day when John puts the medications in the gelatin capsules. It's a game he looks forward to and enjoys.

Occasionally during John's chemotherapy, he experiences bone-marrow depression, evidenced by decreased hemoglobin (9.5) and decreased WBC (<2000). This happens suddenly, and all chemotherapy must be halted until the bone marrow rebuilds itself. During this time, preventing infection is of paramount importance because the white cells are too few to handle the bacteria, and sepsis could occur. John is especially susceptible to skin abscesses during these periods. The first one occurred on his buttocks while he was still wearing diapers, so I bathed him nightly with pHisoHex, rinsing thoroughly. Because John sucked his thumb, it was always wet and a prime target for infection. We tried a pacifier, but John would have none of it. Keeping his thumb dry seemed impossible until we explained that his thumb "is sick" and he must "let it rest and try another finger." Incredibly, he tried very hard to cooperate—partly because the infected finger was too painful to suck. To make sure a second finger didn't become infected, I would examine his fingers every day and put a Band-Aid over a threatening red one. Like most children, John likes Band-Aids, and they helped him remember to try a different finger. During the year, John was content to go from pointer to pinky on either hand. This technique, combined with washing his hands with pHisoHex, ended the finger infections.

Another difficult experience for John was a 12-day period of cobalt therapy (cranial radiation). To be alone, unable to move, beneath a huge machine is enough to frighten an adult; think what it must do to a 2-year-old. We also had to make sure that John lay perfectly still because the beam of scatter radiation fell just above his eyes, and any movement could have caused the rays to damage his eyes, resulting in cataracts in later years.

I explained the whole procedure to John in terms of "having his picture taken," emphasizing that it wouldn't hurt. We took him into the room to see and touch the machine and table before he actually had the therapy. Day number one was the most difficult, but I talked to him constantly through the intercom for the 5-minute treatment. Realizing that we were telling him the truth, that the machine would not harm him, was a great relief to John, but he was still leery.

The next day—and from then on—I brought a few of his favorite books to read to him through the intercom, and this markedly calmed him. As the cobalt timer approached the end of the 5-minute period, I'd tell Johnny to say, "All done, machine," the buzzer would go off, and he was finished. This helped him to personalize the cold metal about him, and seemingly gave him some control over his surroundings. After a few days, John no longer cried when he entered the cobalt room, but jaunted up to the table and tried to climb up by himself.

Two weeks after he'd undergone the cranial radiation, he began to lose his wavy blond hair. I'd anticipated this as a side effect of the radiation and wasn't worried because John was too young to be concerned about his appearance. What I hadn't anticipated was that he would wake up in the morning crying, with hair in his eyes, nose, and mouth. I immediately cut as much of his hair as possible, then put a soft knitted cap on him at night to catch most of the hair. This worked quite well; after 4 days, John was completely bald.

During one period of his chemotherapy, John had a 10-day interim of L-asparaginase therapy. (L-asparaginase is an enzyme which digests the amino acid L-asparagine in the blood. Normal cells can synthesize their own L-asparagine, but leukemic cells cannot.) This drug is given I.V. piggyback, and an infusion had to be started every day for a period of 1 hour in case John had an anaphylactic reaction to the drug. An hour is a long time to ask a 2-year-old to be still, so I again brought books to read to him. Most of all, I relied on an inexpensive plastic slate with a cellophane cover that erases when lifted. This was indispensable and, with a little thought, all kinds of games could be contrived. One that John especially liked was a kind of child's tic-tac-toe. I would first draw a grid on the slate, then draw familiar symbols in random boxes and ask John to point to the triangle, star, or boat. When he identified the symbol correctly, I'd draw the same figure in an adjoining box. Once the slate was filled, we'd change the symbols to owls, cows, cats, and so on. This kept Johnny amused and quiet for the hour—and helped him learn various shapes, too.

Probably the most challenging aspect of Johnny's care has been fostering his trust despite a world of painful, frightening procedures.

In her book, *Nursing Care of the Child With Long-Term Illness,* Shirley Steele questions the common practice of excluding parents when their children are undergoing such procedures. "Certain parents," she says, "could offer much consolation to the child and perhaps even diminish the need for restraining procedures by minimizing the child's fear. Separation of parent and child is an anxiety-producing experience. Each time the child has the procedure done, he should be given a simple, truthful explanation of it. It should not be assumed that the child remembers from the last time or that someone else has prepared him."

Certainly this is how it's worked out for us. Over the course of a year, John has had countless venipunctures. We always tell him ahead of time what is going to happen, then he sits on my lap and we talk about things he likes—airplanes, balloons or something interesting we've seen on our way to the clinic. At the moment of needle penetration, I pull a surprise from a nearby drawer—a 10¢ toy, a piece of candy, sometimes a rock—just anything to distract him.

Of course on days when John doesn't feel well, it's harder, and he often says, "Hide my eyes, Mom." I put my hand over his face so he won't have to see the needle coming. Other times, he *wants* to look. Whenever possible, we allow him some choice in the site of the puncture. Once again, this gives him the feeling of some control over what's happening to him, and reinforces his need for independence that's so strong at this stage of child development. I'm convinced that these small things do reduce his fear and tension, and therefore the pain.

Unfortunately, the bone marrow and lumbar punctures are more painful and frequently John is sedated for these. But we still prepare him by explaining he's going to have a "needle in your back" (LP) or "needle in your bottom" (bone marrow at iliac crest)—phrases that John coined himself, trying to differentiate between the two. We also found that our letting John hold a favorite toy or soft piece of cotton, or just our leaving his little T-shirt on for him to grasp, lets him feel more secure during these procedures.

These, then, are a few practical solutions to some problems that John and I have worked out between us. I hope they might help others in nursing very young children who are seriously ill. My major observation, however—that I want to emphasize—is the need to gain the child's trust. This is the base on which all your nursing care will be built.

As to the personal aspects of being both a mother and nurse of a leukemic child, I feel we've been lucky in one way. Studies show that the major cause of distress in patients under age 6 is separation from the mother. Except for an initial hospitalization of 7 days, that hasn't happened; all of Johnny's care has been as an outpatient. Of course, we can't predict what the future will be, but it's a year now since John was diagnosed leukemic. Every day we have together, Johnny is growing and learning. And so am I. The outlook for this disease is not so bleak as it once was—and we pray.

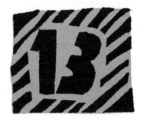

Dorothy Enjoyed Her Reputation as a Mean Old Lady

STELLA K. OLIVER, RN

If you've ever worked in a nursing home, you know how significant the most mundane things can be to your patients, and how important daily routines are. A bingo game becomes an event; dinner, the highlight of the day. Once in a while, though, we find a patient who isn't so taken with routines, who has other ideas about how to spend her time. Dorothy Wilson was such a patient, and in her struggle to keep her independence, she turned our nursing home topsy-turvy.

Dorothy, age 74, was the prototype of the "mean old lady." Cantankerous by nature, unhappy, she'd so alienated all family and friends she had no visitors. Every month, however, she received support money in a plain white envelope with no return address. Part of her cantankerousness, we felt, was a ploy for attention, and because she was so alone, we felt sorry for her. But not as sorry as we might have, because she clearly enjoyed her reputation as an impossible patient and seemed to take a grim satisfaction in defying us.

Dorothy's appearance was as unforgettable as her behavior. Although she had a closet full of clothes, we couldn't get her to change out of a threadbare, polyester pantsuit; an old, peeling pair of pearls; and furry, pink slippers. Always complaining of the cold, she wore thermal underwear, a blouse, and a sweater under her suit, making her look even heavier than her 160 pounds (72 kg). And she always carried a cracked, black plastic purse (circa World War II), which she frequently used as a weapon when we tried to make her do something she didn't feel like doing.

One thing Dorothy didn't feel like doing was having her insulin injection. Every day, she'd postpone her injection as long as possible, stalling for time. She also refused to follow her 2,000-calorie-a-day diabetic diet. Often she'd wait until a senile patient dozed off at dinner, then steal his food and swear to him that he'd eaten it. She also begged for sweets from other patients' visitors, telling them we were starving her.

Needless to say, Dorothy's blood glucose sometimes reached alarming levels, but she had a way of covering this up, too. She'd craftily void only a small amount of urine, then dilute it with water. She also squirreled away medications in her mouth and spat them out when we weren't looking.

On top of all this, Dorothy complained constantly. Her food was either too hot or too cold, her meals either too early or too late, the soap irritated her skin, the toilet paper was too harsh. But Dorothy's pet peeve was her weekly bath. She'd do anything to avoid taking a bath—including calling the police.

One Thursday, a policeman, Sergeant Ambrose, appeared at the door. He was very young, and I could tell he'd never been in a nursing home before.

"You've sure got a lot of old people here," he said, nervously twisting his hat.

I smiled sympathetically. "You're here because of Dorothy Wilson, right?"

"Yes I am, and she has some pretty serious complaints, Miss," the sergeant said.

Taking a notebook from his pocket, he read the complaints: Dorothy was freezing to death, had no blankets on her bed, was starving, and was forced to bathe under inhuman conditions.

Of course, none of these complaints was justified, and wanting to show the sergeant just how well we cared for our patients, I took the long way to Dorothy's room. I hoped he would notice how clean, fresh-smelling, and homey our facility was. On the way, I explained the situation to him.

"Thursday is Dorothy's bath day," I said, "and every week she tries to get out of bathing. When she can't, she takes matters into her own hands. One Thursday she called the fire department with a false alarm. When the commotion finally died down, we'd *forgotten* about her bath."

Sergeant Ambrose looked disbelieving. "I never heard of anyone who hated bathing that much."

When I opened the door to Dorothy's room, a warm blast of air hit me. The thermostat was set at 85° F. (29.4° C.), and Dorothy's note above it read: "If you touch this, I'll break your fingers." I turned back the bed covers and counted 10 blankets. The sergeant gaped and mopped his forehead with a handkerchief.

"I see what you mean," he said, "but I still have to talk to Mrs. Wilson."

I told him he could talk with her privately in the chapel, and as I closed the chapel door on the sergeant and Dorothy, I felt a bit guilty. Dorothy hadn't had a bath in 2 weeks, and the small chapel was windowless.

When the sergeant found me later at the nurses' station, he was visibly shaken. "It was, uh, stuffy in there," he said, "and she sure talked my ear off."

Then, professional again, he asked me to sign Dorothy's list of complaints—it was required. By now, I knew the routine.

"We're required to drop in unannounced to investigate these charges," he said—but his heart wasn't in it.

"Try to come on a Thursday," I said.

That afternoon, when I arrived to give Dorothy her bath, she was lying in bed under 10 blankets, wiping her nose with a large, gray handkerchief.

"I think I'm coming down with a cold," she said, sneezing and blowing her nose.

I took her temperature, pulse, and blood pressure—all normal. "You're fine, Dorothy," I said, "and you're getting your bath." We launched into our foreordained battle of wills, with Dorothy shouting and calling me names. That night, her complaints reached a crescendo, and the night shift bore the brunt of her tirade. Wide-awake and high on anger, Dorothy threw the unit into a turmoil.

At breakfast the next morning, she sent her entire meal back to the kitchen, and when the new meal didn't meet with her approval, she threw it on the floor. At lunch, she threw a dish of pudding at a nurse, and the nurse burst into tears.

We were at wit's end, and I decided on a course of action that, God willing, might improve Dorothy's behavior. Unpleasant as it might be, I'd take full responsibility for Dorothy for the next week (including the next bath day). If she wanted attention, I'd give her attention. I'd follow her around like a handmaiden; I'd be cheerful, sympathetic, and solicitous. (This would also give me a chance to monitor her food intake and make sure she didn't sabotage her urine tests.) Hopefully, Dorothy would start behaving better just to get me off her back. In short, I'd try to be as devious as she was.

I started my campaign the next morning. "How are you today, Dorothy? Isn't it a lovely day?" I asked.

Her suspicions were aroused immediately. "What are you so happy about?" she snapped. "How am I? I'm terrible; I'm getting pneumonia because I took a bath in this freezing room."

I patted her arm sympathetically and reassured

her that she wasn't getting pneumonia. Then I prepared her insulin injection. "This will only take a second," I said.

Pouting, with her upper lip trembling in anger, Dorothy went into her usual pre-injection routine. Standing in the corner and glowering like a trapped animal, she slowly, ever so slowly, rolled up the sleeves of her jacket, sweater, blouse, and thermal underwear.

"Ready?" I asked.

"Wait, this arm's too sore," she said.

Trying not to think about the dozen other injections and the two trays of crushed medications I still had to give, I watched as Dorothy slowly rolled down her sleeves and even more slowly rolled up the sleeves on her other arm. She yelled "ouch" before I even touched her with the needle.

"There, there, that wasn't so bad, was it?" I said soothingly.

"Hurt like hell and you know it," she snapped.

After I finished giving out medications, Dorothy got my undivided attention for the rest of the day. And during the rest of the week, I was always there to "help." I followed Dorothy into the bathroom and personally collected her urine specimens. Anticipating her every move, I waited until she was at dinner and then searched her room, removing a cache of forbidden foods. Dorothy was furious, but we were finally getting accurate results from her fasting blood sugar test.

For the first few days, Dorothy hit me with her usual barrage of complaints. I made soothing noises—even encouraged her—and found that if I kept her busy talking, I could pop her pills in her mouth and she'd swallow them without missing a syllable. After a few more days, though, Dorothy got tired of my almost constant presence.

"You're gettin' on my nerves," she grumbled. "Don't you have something else to do?"

"My job is to keep you happy and healthy," I said, groaning inwardly.

"Someone told the nurses on the other floors I was stealing food off the carts." She eyed me accusingly. "I can be mean when I'm crossed, you know."

I knew. With effort, I smiled and said, "I'm only trying to do something about your dissatisfactions. That's why I'm spending so much time with you."

"You're overdoing it," Dorothy said.

As Dorothy's next bath day approached, I planned it as carefully as the Normandy invasion. On Thursday afternoon, while Dorothy watched television in the lounge, I turned the thermostat in her room up to 85° F. (29.4° C.), threw her flannel nightgown and robe in the washer, stripped her bed and washed the linens, and put her robe in the dryer so it would be nice and warm after her bath. Then I ran hot water in the tub to steam up the bathroom, and went to get Dorothy.

She knew what was coming, and she was prepared, too. When we got to her room, she folded her arms across her chest and said, "I'm not taking off my clothes and you're not touching me."

"If you'd just cooperate, Dorothy, we could get this over with in no time," I said.

"Why should I cooperate—you don't," she said. "Why did you steal all my goodies?"

"I didn't. I just cut down on the appropriation of food that wasn't yours. Now you're getting only the food you're allowed," I said.

"Well, I'm starving, and you're pretty mean," she said.

"No I'm not, Dorothy. I've just been watching you and I'm on to your little games," I said.

As we talked, I removed Dorothy's clothing piece by piece, and she was so caught up in our conversation that I had her almost completely undressed—except for her thermal underwear and purse.

"Look what you've done, you sneak," Dorothy yelled, stamping her foot like a child. Then she swung her purse and missed my head by inches.

Now my knees were trembling. "I'm not leaving until you've had a bath," I said, edging around the tub to put some space between me and that purse. I kept up a steady stream of conversation.

"You twit!" Dorothy yelled, swinging her purse again. This time, it flew from her hands and hit the wall with a smack, spewing sugar and salt packets, candy, and crushed cookies. I couldn't believe it. After all my careful watching, Dorothy was still getting forbidden foods and hiding them in the one place I dared not violate.

"Dor-o-thy!" I said, letting my anger show for the first time.

Incredibly, Dorothy's anger dissipated as fast as mine had flared. She meekly removed her underwear, took my arm, and stepped gingerly into the tub. As the water covered most of her body, she shrieked, "You're shrinking me," and I couldn't help but think of the Wicked Witch of the West, who'd melted when water was thrown on her.

I finished Dorothy's bath that day with a minimum of trouble. And during the next few weeks, she was unusually subdued. She grumbled rather than complained, and she ate what was put in front of her. Her purse was empty of goodies, and she actually lost a few pounds. Her blood glucose level was almost normal. Everyone thought I'd worked a miracle, but I wasn't convinced. The Dorothys of this world don't give up that easily.

A month later, when warm spring rains gave us the first taste of summer and beckoned us all to seize the moment—Dorothy did. When she failed to show up for breakfast, and we couldn't find her anywhere on the unit, we sent out a general alarm to all floors. No Dorothy. She was gone, all right, and I, better than anyone, knew why. Her reputation as a stubborn, cranky old woman was at stake, and determined to keep that reputation and some semblance of independence, she'd run away.

But to where? She had no friends that we knew of, and her relatives weren't giving out their address. Someone remembered seeing a cab parked in front of the building that morning. So we called the police, and 2 hours later, they located the cab driver. He remembered Dorothy well.

"She asked me to drive her to a pancake house," he said, "and then she invited me to have breakfast with her. Wow. Never saw an old lady eat so much. Then she excused herself to go to the ladies' room, and never came back. She left without paying her fare, and stuck me with her breakfast check."

That was Dorothy, for sure, but where was she now? I kept busy with charts and orders, but I couldn't shake the feeling that I was partly responsible for Dorothy's disappearance. My co-workers were sympathetic—of course it wasn't my fault. I'd done so much for Dorothy. Still, I wondered—how far did my responsibility go? Maybe Dorothy's health was as much her responsibility as mine. My thoughts about her rights as an individual were all mixed up with my feelings about my role as a nurse.

I stayed long after my shift ended, waiting for news. Then at 9 p.m., in a driving rainstorm, the police escorted a wet, disheveled Dorothy through the door. They'd found her in a bus station 10 miles (16 km) away. I was so glad to see her, I could've kissed her.

"How could you turn an old lady like me out in the rain?" Dorothy said, looking me square in the eye.

That night, Dorothy submitted to a hot bath without a fuss. But she refused to tell us what had happened to her that day, or what she'd been doing at a bus station. For weeks after, though, she refused to go outside at all.

We continued to monitor Dorothy's diet closely, but because we knew how important her little games were to her, we gave her the liberty of trying to con visitors into bringing her food—never letting her get too much. She still stole food occasionally, and we allowed her to eat forbidden foods on holidays and other special occasions. Bath time was never easy, but we managed. And there were no more phone calls to the police or fire department.

Dorothy's complaints remained constant and legendary, I do have to admit. But we realized that, in some perverse way, it was her responsibility to complain, her way of getting attention, of having some control over her life, some independence. Old habits die hard—for nurses as well as patients. And we all must make compromises.

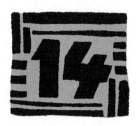

Sam Was Dying.…We Had to Help Him Live Again

JOYCE EDDY, RN
ROSEMARIE SELGAS CORDES, RN, MSN
MARILYN CURRAN, RN, BSN

What kind of hope can we offer to a dying patient? Most of us have asked ourselves this question, but the answer doesn't come easy—especially to those of us who work with dying patients almost exclusively.

For 4 years, we've been involved in a research project on mycosis fungoides—an uncommon, often fatal form of cutaneous T-cell lymphoma. We've cared for more than 70 patients with this disease, and although we haven't found a cure, we *have* been able to add months, even years, to some patients' lives, and also improve the quality of their lives. Sam was one of these patients.

Sam, 27 years old, had had skin diseases all his life. As a child he'd had eczema, which caused him social embarrassment and rejection. After high school, he'd joined the army, but was medically discharged because of bleeding skin lesions on his thighs. Later, working in a carpet factory, his skin became so irritated by dyes and glues that he was forced to quit his job. Finally, he was treated at a hospital near his hometown, where the diagnosis of mycosis fungoides was made. Sam's hometown hospital referred him to us.

The first thing we noticed about Sam was that, although he did have facial tumors and skin lesions, he wasn't as badly disfigured as some of our patients. The next thing we noticed was that Sam laughed and joked right from the start. Frankly, we were a little afraid that he wouldn't take us seriously when we explained the tests he'd have to undergo—he didn't even seem to take *himself* very seriously, because he was carrying a fuzzy red teddy bear.

Sam explained that the bear, "Buggish," was a going-away gift from Della, his wife—a substitute traveling companion since she and his two young sons couldn't be with him.

We told Sam about all the tests he'd be having—biopsies of his skin, lymph nodes, bone marrow, and liver, and a liver scan, peritoneoscopy, and lymphangiogram. He listened to our explanations closely and was very cooperative during the tests. Unfortunately, the tests showed that Sam had stage IV B mycosis fungoides—the disease had spread to his lymph nodes and to the bones in his left foot, and the doctors felt Sam wouldn't live more than a year. The only treatment at this stage was chemotherapy and radiotherapy, so we asked Sam to return once a week for these treatments.

When Sam learned of his poor prognosis, he cried, saying, "Why me?" over and over. Although we'd witnessed this reaction many times with other patients, we never got used to it. How can you comfort a patient who has, maybe, a year to live?

We gave Sam all the support we could, hoping that he'd be able to accept his death. And unbelievably, Sam snapped out of his depression quickly, and was soon joking and laughing again. He was sharing a room with three sickly, elderly men, and peals of laughter began echoing from the once-gloomy room. We were relieved. Perhaps, after years of illness, Sam had been *prepared* for his prognosis.

Sam was discharged after 2 days, and he returned to his home, 1,000 miles away. The research grant covered all his travel expenses, and once a week he came to our hospital for chemotherapy and radiotherapy. Buggish went everywhere with him and was a real icebreaker. On planes, in the hospital, whenever Sam felt anxious or insecure, he resorted to Buggish jokes. The bear seemed almost like Sam's alter ego.

Chemotherapy and radiotherapy helped clear up Sam's facial tumors and kept the disease under control for 8 months. But then one day at home, Sam was playing with one of his sons, and the child accidentally stepped hard on Sam's foot. An ulcer developed at the site of the injury, and because of the disease, the ulcer wouldn't heal.

We did our best to keep Sam an outpatient, because we knew how much he wanted to be with his family. So we taught him to do wet-to-dry dressing changes. He'd wet fine-mesh gauze with saline, apply the gauze to the wound, and then cover the gauze with Cling so when he removed the dry dressing, he'd debride the wound. We also explained the procedure to Della over the phone.

But after several months with no improvement, we wondered how well Sam and Della were following our directions. From past experience, we figured they were probably wetting the dressing before they removed it, so the procedure wouldn't be so painful. Now we had no choice—Sam had to be admitted to the hospital.

Sam agreed to hospitalization reluctantly, but

nevertheless in good humor. Of course, Buggish was installed beside him in bed. But after only one day, we began to notice a drastic change in Sam. He became very lethargic, his eyes looked vacant, and he didn't recognize any of us.

The doctors did a lumbar puncture and found that abnormal lymphocytes had entered Sam's cerebrospinal fluid. He went into surgery immediately, and an Ommaya shunt was inserted into the ventricles of his brain. The shunt provided a way for chemotherapeutic drugs (which don't cross the blood-brain barrier) to be injected into Sam's brain through a catheter.

Sam received dexamethasone (Decadron) and methotrexate through the shunt, and also had cranial irradiation. Fortunately, his mental status returned to normal after a few days. But no sooner was one problem solved than another presented itself. Sam's foot ulcer got larger, with more necrotic tissue. We began a program of even more intense ulcer care, but as the weeks passed, we all knew amputation was inevitable.

Sam panicked, adamantly refusing even to consider amputation. Suddenly, all his fears came to the surface. We understood what he was going through—he'd been plagued with illness since childhood, yet had managed to live a comparatively normal life. Now, the disease he'd struggled with for so long and had learned to accept had gotten the better of him.

Sam became more and more listless. Many mornings we'd find him sitting motionless, staring at the washcloth and towel, unable to perform even the simplest tasks. He also began resisting getting out of bed, and we ended up taking over just about all of his personal care as he gradually lost interest in doing anything.

Except crying—which he did frequently and loudly. This upset Sam's roommates terribly and upset us just as much. We tried to spend some time each day talking with Sam, but these visits became so emotionally draining and seemed so fruitless that we found ourselves deliberately avoiding him—even taking a different hallway so we wouldn't have to pass his room. But if we did happen to rush by, Sam would *beg* us to just call out a greeting if we couldn't stop to visit.

Naturally, we couldn't go on like this, so we asked the psychiatric nurse for advice. She told us to sit with Sam and let him cry—that this was what he needed most. And although it was one of the hardest things we ever did, we spent countless hours just holding Sam's hand while he cried.

Still, we felt this wasn't enough. We searched for ways to pull Sam out of his depression, to give him enough hope in the future so that he might at least consent to the amputation.

First, we used Buggish. Focusing attention on the funny red bear helped resurrect Sam's sense of humor. When an alert lab technician noticed Buggish's stuffing falling out, she performed "emergency surgery" with a needle and thread on Buggish's "liver." At least that made Sam smile.

Then one day Buggish disappeared. We staged an all-out search, alerting practically the whole hospital, including the janitors. Sam was really upset—but even he had to laugh about the search. Two days later, a janitor found the bear wedged between the mattress frame and side rail of Sam's bed. At least the episode was a welcome distraction.

We also tried appealing to Sam's religious beliefs, since he and Della were devout Christians. One of us got Sam a Bible, and we often sat with him while he read and prayed aloud. We thought, too, that Sam needed a constructive outlet for his depression, so we brought him a notebook and encouraged him to keep a diary of all the things he was feeling and experiencing.

But probably the biggest source of comfort to Sam was Della—he loved her intensely. Since their financial situation prevented Della from visiting or even calling often, we tried to get Sam to talk about her. This never failed to raise his spirits.

Our efforts helped some, but not enough. Sam continued to refuse amputation. Then he did something totally out of character. He began capitalizing on a rift that had developed between the clinic nurses and the staff nurses. The clinic nurses, who'd known Sam as a jovial outpatient, still visited him and were deeply sympathetic. Of course, the staff nurses were sympathetic, too, but with Sam's demanding care schedule and increasingly dependent behavior, they were also straining to control their impatience with him. Antagonistic feelings soon developed between the two factions.

Sam saw this happening and took advantage of the situation, reporting to the clinic nurses that the staff nurses were "unkind." So to head off unprofessional confrontations, we held a short staff conference and managed to straighten things out. Then we had the psychiatric nurse talk to Sam about his behavior. Sam, deeply offended, pleaded innocent—but his manipulative behavior stopped.

Meanwhile, his condition was deteriorating rapidly. Besides everything else, his vision began to blur until he could scarcely recognize us. The doctors felt that the visual problem was probably temporary—a side effect of the radiotherapy. So we told Sam this, and then prayed that the doctors were right.

As Sam's problems multiplied, he resisted amputation with even more fervor. But now the foot ulcer was beginning to smell more and more foul. Room deodorizers no longer helped. Sam's roommates started taking their meal trays into the lounge and also began complaining that Sam's loud crying was keeping them awake at night.

Matters reached an all-time low one morning when one of Sam's roommates said that Sam had flung feces from his bedpan onto his roommate's bed. Sam denied it, claiming it was an accident. But now Sam would have to move to a private room—leaving him where he was would be unfair to the other patients. We worried that Sam would interpret this as the ultimate rejection and become even more depressed, and we discussed this at a team conference, vowing to make an extra effort to spend more "social" time with Sam.

As we feared, the move was devastating to him. He became even more withdrawn, and spent most days with his head buried under the sheets.

Finally, we decided that if we couldn't reach Sam, maybe the person he loved most could. So we thought of a way to have Della flown to the hospital.

We asked the hospital administrator if we could use money from a special fund for needy patients. She agreed, so the arrangements were made posthaste. When Della arrived, we bent the rules a bit and installed a pullout sofa for her in Sam's room.

The tiny woman took command immediately. She was so composed, so dignified, and she never seemed put off by Sam's disease. Frequently, she'd lie in bed next to him, and we'd try to leave them alone as long as we could.

Della stayed a month. During her visit, Sam's

vision improved and gradually returned to normal. And by the end of the month, Della had somehow convinced Sam to have his foot amputated. The doctors scheduled him for surgery.

Once Sam had made this decision, we felt an incredible peace descend upon us. The strain of caring for Sam and watching his disease progress had caused such tension among all of us. We held our breath, hardly daring to hope (but hoping nonetheless) that once the surgery was over, Sam would be his old self again.

Sam's surgery went well, and in the days that followed, he actually seemed anxious to get on with his life. He felt better, and although Della had to return home, he was confident he'd be joining her soon. Now he looked forward to physical therapy, and diligently practiced transferring himself from bed to wheelchair. We brought him a large calendar and printed his daily schedule on it; from then on, he took full responsibility for getting himself to physical therapy. He progressed rapidly and was soon a candidate for a prosthesis.

We were so relieved by this change in Sam and so happy that the ordeal was over that we focused all our efforts on his rehabilitation as an amputee. We almost—but not quite—forgot that his disease was still there, because every time we thought, *Sam's still dying,* it was like a slap in the face.

Perhaps we were denying, too, but pushing Sam's death into the back of our minds probably helped us rehabilitate him more quickly.

We conducted role-playing sessions with him, acting out his return home and trying to anticipate reactions from his family and friends. We explained that if his children were curious, he should encourage them to look at and feel his stump, and we brought him a book detailing the accomplishments and adjustments of amputees.

After 4 months' hospitalization, Sam returned home, and 1 month later, he returned to the hospital for final prosthetic fittings. He proudly showed us a photograph of Della and him at an awards ceremony for the basketball team he was coaching. The smiles on their faces and the crutches in the background testified to Sam's adjustment.

But when we entered his room this time, we noticed something missing.

"Where's Buggish?" we asked.

Sam grinned as he explained that Buggish hadn't come because he'd fallen in love with a little pink panda. And although Sam had lost his traveling companion, he'd regained what he needed desperately—his sense of humor and his enthusiasm for living.

Rose Demanded a Special Kind of Love

CATHERINE YORK, RN

I used to think that love came in only one size, color, and texture: large, pink, and fuzzy. Well, I was wrong. There's another kind of love called Tough Love. It's cut from coarser material.

You've probably heard of Tough Love before—it works miracles for motivating troubled teenagers. But Tough Love for a nursing-home resident? I'd never considered it...not before 92-year-old Rose LaPointe arrived at our retirement home. She taught me the importance of balancing compassion with firmness when caring for elderly patients like her. That's Tough Love.

From the day she was admitted, Rose was a showstopper. Wheeled into the lobby in the biggest, reddest wheelchair I'd ever seen, she looked like a deposed queen still ensconced on her throne. She seemed utterly disgusted and bored.

As her middle-aged daughter guided her down the hallway toward the administrator's office, Rose caught my eye. As if by magic, the wheelchair rolled to a stop. A stubby finger shot up and wiggled a friendly "come here." Smiling, I bent down close to her so I'd be able to hear. And hear her I did.

"Life's a lot of garbage, honey," she said pointedly. "And looking at this joint, I can see where it all gets dumped." I'm not sure what my face was expressing at that instant, but she laughed so loudly that some hearing-impaired residents in the activity room poked their heads into the hallway. Her daughter turned bright red and whispered, "You'll have to forgive my mother."

Forgive her? I could hardly *believe* her. She'd been inside the home less than a minute and she'd already declared it a dump.

Like our 75 residents, the staff was proud of our retirement home. For us, it was a place of serenity and order set in a rural community amidst rich, rolling farmland. Mainly churchgoers from nearby small towns, our residents were pleasant, polite, and quiet. Besides all that, our home was clean and cheery. How could this newcomer say such a crude thing?

We soon realized that Rose took pride in saying other crude things. And the more unexpected they were, the more delighted she became. Almost automatically, my ears would perk up as she'd come down the hall in her oversized wheelchair. When somebody would greet her with a spirited, "God bless you," she'd quickly reply, "Stick it in your ear." And that wasn't even Rose at her worst. She'd wait to throw her juiciest epithets around in the evening when families were visiting.

There was still more. When she wasn't wheeling herself to the dining hall or physical therapy (PT) room, she'd retreat to her own room where she'd either lie in bed or sit in her wheelchair, refusing to talk to anyone.

Then suddenly she'd become animated in her own special way. She was what you might call an aggressive flirt. Patiently, she'd wait inside the doorway of her room until an unsuspecting male resident passed by. Then, working the wheels of her chair with lightning-fast reflexes, she'd spring out at him, cutting him off in midstride. She'd say something provocative and personal and then wait for a reaction.

She always got one. Mostly embarrassment.

She liked testing everybody's limits. "Making headlines" is the way she put it to me. Putting it to the whole staff, we soon realized, was her way of interrupting the overwhelming predictability of institutional living. A self-satisfied belly laugh was her release valve. And one of her trademarks.

But soon we'd had enough of one of her other trademarks, her foul language. Our first challenge was to sweeten her sour mouth. Talking politely to Rose about it did no good. Even the psychiatric counselor got a hot earful from her. But one night after she'd verbally abused one of our aides, I marched into her room. I was angry with her. And I told her so. "Now, Rose, here's where we start drawing lines," I said, watching her inch back and forth in her wheelchair.

I explained that any time she became loud or aggressive in the home, she'd be taken back to her room, where she'd stay until she apologized. As simple and direct as my warning was, it worked. During the next few months, I noticed a marked improvement in her speech. No one was more surprised than I was.

I learned an important lesson from that experience: Being direct and firm with Rose was the only way to get her attention. Be meek, and she'd walk all over you. Now I had to apply that lesson to another problem. I'm talking about her big, red wheelchair.

"My doctor tells me that a woman my age deserves to live the rest of her life in a wheelchair, being waited on hand and foot," she said. And believe me, she took her doctor's advice literally. For the first 6 months with us, she refused to get out of it except to go to bed. So one day when I saw her doctor, I explained what I thought. That wheelchair was a dual symbol for Rose, I said. In one way, it was a positive symbol. It meant security. And since her wheelchair was distinctly different from all the other wheelchairs in our nursing home, it reinforced the idea that she was an individual. That was good for her.

But the wheelchair was a negative influence, too. It was an excuse for her... an excuse to avoid becoming more mobile and independent, to limit

 She was what you might call an aggressive flirt. Patiently, she'd wait inside her doorway until an unsuspecting male resident passed by. Then, working the wheels of her chair with lightning speed, she'd spring out at him, cutting him off in midstride. She'd say something provocative and personal and then wait for a reaction.

her interactions with other residents in the activity room, to even stop *trying*. Clearly, her unhealthy attachment to the wheelchair had to be broken.

But how? After talking with her doctor, I resolved to shift her out of the wheelchair and onto a walker. I'd do it gradually. First, I allowed her to use the chair to get from her room to the PT room, about 100 feet (30 meters) down the hall. Once there, though, she'd have to transfer to a walker or one of our standard gray wheelchairs. The choice was hers, but under no circumstances was the big, red wheelchair allowed in PT.

The second step, which I implemented 2 weeks later, was to ban the chair completely from her room, while limiting the amount of time she could stay in bed. That encouraged her to spend more time with others. She could use the walker to move from her bed to the bathroom and to the hallway, where her chair was stationed.

The next step was the toughest. She was permitted to ride from her room to PT only in a standard wheelchair. The red wheelchair stayed in the activity room where she could sit (but not ride) in it whenever she liked. Now she had to use the walker in her room and in the PT room, and to get from the hallway to her wheelchair in the activity room.

Predictably, she resisted this change, complaining that her feet hurt too much for her to walk so frequently. She threw temper tantrums, too. The

 Being direct and firm with Rose was the only way to get her attention. Be meek, and she'd walk all over you. "My doctor tells me that a woman my age deserves to live the rest of her life in a wheelchair, being waited on hand and foot," she said.

cleaning woman once fled the activity room in tears when Rose accused her of daring to touch the red wheelchair. Rose spent an entire afternoon in her room until she finally apologized.

Progress with her was slow. For a few days, I even considered letting Rose continue to use her wheelchair. But then I remembered how much more she respected a firm attitude than a lax one. So I bore down on her. Week by week, I made sure she exercised her legs more. After 3 months of my coaching, she was able to make it anywhere in the home using only a walker. She complained bitterly every step of the way. But she did it.

I knew I'd finally broken her dependence on her wheelchair when we were able to store it in the basement.

Now that she was out of the wheelchair and using a walker, I realized that her walking problems were partly caused by her shoes—cracked patent leather, circa 1961. For the past 6 months, she'd refused to replace them with new shoes. Then one evening while she was soaking her feet in Epsom salts, I poked my head into her room. "New shoes would sure help make walking easier, Rose. Don't you think it's time?" I said. Reluctantly, she finally agreed.

So the next morning, I brought her a new pair. They were brown walking shoes, and I'll never forget the look on her face as I helped her try them on for size. "I always hated brown shoes," she said. "Brown shoes look just like cow sh—."

"That's enough, Rose," I said. "Let's try walking in them."

Rose walked as far as the lobby before she decided she'd had enough. Suddenly letting go of my arm, she sat down in the middle of the floor and tried to pull off her new shoes. "Brown...yuck," she kept repeating as her arthritic fingers struggled with the laces.

That's when I made a mistake. Instead of speaking to her sternly, I pleaded with her to get up. Disliking any show of weakness, she ignored me. Then Mrs. Murphy, our administrator, spotted Rose. With eyes narrowing, she ordered her to get to her feet and come into the conference room. Rose did. *Immediately.*

As the door closed, I just stood there. First I heard one voice, declarative and strong. Then I heard a second voice, a lot less sure of itself. Then the first voice again, even stronger this time.

Two minutes later, the door opened and Mrs. Murphy walked out, somewhat breathless but with a determined look. After a few more seconds, Rose shuffled out, wearing the brown shoes. Catching sight of me in the hallway, she pulled herself together quickly. She turned toward the vanishing figure of Mrs. Murphy. And after prudently clearing her throat, she declared as matter-of-factly as she could, "Thanks for the little chat, Mrs. Murphy. We must do this again sometime."

No, nothing was ever easy with Rose. She wasn't cut out of the same mold as our other residents. But that didn't mean she wasn't a part of their lives. Sure, she wasn't always sweet or gentle. And she certainly wasn't a churchgoer. But she wasn't vicious, either. Sometimes she could show an almost maternal tenderness toward the other residents. Usually, if she was going to stick it to somebody, she'd pick on a staff member.

Once, when one of our newer residents complained about the exercise bicycle in PT, I overheard Rose—a physical therapy veteran—encourage her. "I know how you feel," she said softly. "It'll be all right if you listen to the nurses. Just don't tell them I told you that." Naturally, she didn't want anybody else to hear her. It wouldn't be good for her image as a tough little old lady.

And in her own way, she was kind to the men in the home, too: Her flirting flattered them. And you know what? Sometimes I'd notice a little flicker of jealousy on some of the women's faces. You could hardly blame them. Rose did exactly what many of them might like to do. She was...well, *direct*. If she had something to say, she'd say it. You knew exactly where you stood.

There wasn't a trace of false advertising about her.

All this became very clear to me a few months after we'd put her wheelchair in the basement. One of our residents, Mr. Samuelson, a diabetic leg amputee, asked me if he could borrow Rose's old red wheelchair since she wasn't using it anymore. He thought it was "snazzy" and wanted to use it until he was fitted with a prosthesis. I said, "Let's find out, shall we? Come on, we'll ask Rose." I doubted she'd loan it to him, though.

When we asked, her eyes closed and the corners of her mouth dropped. She almost looked as if she were going to cry. When she said, "Take it if you want it so bad. I sure as hell don't need it now," Mr. Samuelson's face lit up. And so did mine. I could have kissed her.

Later, I found her alone in her room, and I touched her shoulder. "That was very sweet of you to lend Mr. Samuelson your wheelchair. I know what it means to you," I said. She looked up at me, and for an instant I thought she was going to say something nice. But then her face shifted gears. She said, "Ah, stick it in your—"

"*Rose*."

"I'm sorry...."

Tough Love means sometimes having to say you're sorry. It means making sure your patients take responsibility for their actions and words, and that isn't always easy, depending on which patients you're caring for. For independent and willful older people like Rose LaPointe, Tough Love may be the only kind of love they can take, because it's the only kind they can give.

By Losing Control of Herself, Linda Controlled Her Parents...and Us

BEVERLY Z. FARO, RN, MS

When children are seriously ill, their parents tend to make them the center of attention. But over-indulging children only compounds their problems—no one knows this better than pediatric nurses, who have to care for these children.

Eight-year-old Linda Foster had been in and out of hospitals all her life, and she was *angry*. And although we couldn't blame Linda for being angry, we had to control her screaming and crying—for her sake, her parents', and our own.

Linda was admitted to our pediatric unit for surgical correction of scoliosis and lordosis—problems so severe she'd never walk without braces and crutches. Shortly after her admission, she'd had an anterior cervical spinal fusion and was scheduled for a posterior spinal fusion and insertion of a Harrington rod in 3 weeks. Besides her orthopedic problems, Linda had other birth defects—a T-12 myelomeningocele, which had been repaired at birth, and hydrocephalus, which had been corrected at infancy by a ventriculoperitoneal shunt.

Linda's home was a 4-hour drive from the hospital, so Mr. and Mrs. Foster stayed with Linda for several days after her surgery. But even though her parents were always close by, Linda couldn't bear to have them out of her sight. Every time they left her room, she'd cry violently—and the longer they were gone, the louder she cried. The Fosters, obviously embarrassed by Linda's outbursts, rarely left her room, even for meals.

The Fosters had three other children, so 5 days after Linda's surgery, they left for home, promising to visit every weekend. Linda cried and begged them to stay. And after they were gone, her cries turned to screams. The only thing that kept her from having a full-fledged temper tantrum—complete with kicking—was the posterior shell she wore, which limited her movement.

At first the posterior shell seemed a blessing in disguise—it kept Linda from acting out violently. But before long, the staff realized it created more problems than it solved. Linda seemed to use the shell as an excuse for not doing anything for herself. She refused to perform even the simplest tasks, like brushing her teeth or washing her face, and her demands for attention were incessant. If the nurses didn't respond to her buzzer immediately, she threw a tantrum, and when they tried to change her dressing or give her an injection, she became hysterical.

Fortunately, I seemed to be in the right place at the right time. As a graduate student, one of my assignments was doing play therapy with long-term patients. Linda seemed an ideal patient.

When I first met Linda, she was lying passively in bed, her small, chubby body encased in the posterior shell. She seemed frightened by my approach, but when I told her we were just going to talk, she relaxed and smiled shyly. The surgery for her hydrocephalus had apparently been successful, because her head was normal sized. But something about her demeanor bothered me, and I knew it bothered the other nurses, too. Linda's violent behavior—her hysteria, screaming, and temper tantrums—seemed inappropriate for an 8-year-old.

I suspected that Linda's floor charts didn't tell the whole story. So since I had more time than the other nurses, I looked for Linda's old charts in our outpatient birth defects clinic. In them, I discovered a possible explanation for some of her problem behavior. Linda's I.Q. was 85, and tests showed developmental delays in several areas.

Linda's records also listed the name of a public health nurse who'd cared for her. I called the nurse, and she told me that Linda'd been in a special school for retarded children for 3 years, but that this year she was enrolled in the first grade of a public school. The nurse also said that Mr. Foster worked in a factory and most of the Fosters' financial and emotional resources were spent meeting Linda's needs.

My first goal was to make Linda's separation from her family more tolerable for everyone, including Linda. I hoped that I could help her learn to express her anger in constructive ways, instead of resorting to temper tantrums. I also hoped that by letting her "play nurse" with a doll and hospital equipment, I could help her adjust to hospitalization and prepare her for her second surgery.

Our unit has a full-time play director, so Linda'd been to the playroom before. Understandably, the play director didn't always have time to give individual attention, but *I* had time to give Linda 3 hours of undivided attention a week and make her playtime a *learning* time as well.

During our first play session, I gave Linda an anesthesia mask, a nurse's operating room mask and cap, syringes without needles, sponges, forceps, and I.V. equipment. I also gave her books and toys. At first, I used nondirective play with Linda—I simply let her do her own thing. And during our first play session, she played nurse with a doll.

 Eight-year-old Linda Foster had been in and out of hospitals all her life, and she was angry. And although we couldn't blame Linda for being angry, we had to control her screaming and crying—for her sake, her parents', and our own.

The more I worked with Linda, the more obvious her learning disabilities became—although differentiating between what Linda *couldn't* and *wouldn't* do wasn't always easy. She had a short attention span, and lost interest in most games quickly. Her visual-motor coordination was poor, so she had trouble drawing pictures and putting together puzzles. And she couldn't talk about past experiences without a great deal of reinforcement. For instance, she couldn't discuss her last operation unless I gave her a doll and an anesthesia mask.

Linda also had little concept of time, so she asked the same questions over and over, like: "When's lunch?" or "When's my mother coming?"

I wanted to help Linda understand the passage of time as it related to her hospital routine. First, I made a large cardboard calendar with squares for each day of the month. I pasted pictures in the squares to represent important events—toys on days I'd be playing with her, snapshots of her parents on days they'd be visiting, and a surgical mask on the day of her next operation. I taped the calendar next to her bed, so she could draw an "X" through each day. Every time Linda asked about a future event, I'd point to the calendar and count the days with her.

Next, I made a cardboard clock with movable hands. Then, I pasted pictures of daily routines—vital sign checks, meals, baths—on cards, and stacked the cards in order of occurrence. Every morning Linda'd look through her cards and have a picture of what would be happening next, and when.

I thought role-playing with puppets might also be an effective device to use with Linda—and to a certain extent, it was. Linda loved the puppets, but she was rather ritualistic in her role-playing—acting out the same scenes over and over. Occasionally, though, she let her anger show. Sometimes she'd make the puppets "cry," and once, she told me she thought her parents loved her brothers more than her.

Whenever Linda showed her anger in a constructive way, I congratulated her. "I'm glad you told me that, Linda," I'd say. "You know, lots of kids get mad at their parents, even though they're very glad to see them." Still, Linda never admitted she was angry at her parents, only that she missed them.

I decided to try role-playing with Linda's parents, too, when they visited that weekend. I hoped that if I played the part of Linda and asked them to respond in their usual way, they'd see how she was manipulating them.

Then I had another idea. Since the Fosters could afford only one brief phone call a week, I'd borrow a tape recorder for them, so they could record family dinner conversations for Linda to play when she was lonely.

I called the Fosters, and they said they were more than happy to record their conversations. In fact, they were so anxious to try the idea that *they* decided to borrow the tape recorder and tape some conversations before their next visit.

I made a point to be nearby when the Fosters visited and asked them to call me if things got tough. And things *did* get tough. When Linda saw her parents she was ecstatic, hugging and kissing them, clinging to her mother. But when the Fosters

mentioned they were going to the cafeteria for lunch, Linda screamed so much, they ate lunch in her room. When they told her they were leaving in an hour, Linda crossed her arms, pouted, and refused to look at them. Then, for lack of a more appropriate response, Mrs. Foster said, "Linda, if you don't talk to us, we're leaving right now."

"I hate you," Linda screamed.

At this point, the Fosters called me into the room and told me what'd happened. They said it'd taken them an hour just to get out of Linda's room last time—that her crying was breaking their hearts. They were overcome with guilt and emotionally exhausted. What could they do?

I wanted to be completely honest with the Fosters, but I had to be tactful. After all, their relationship with their daughter was a highly emotional subject, and I didn't want to alienate them.

I told the Fosters that they had to set limits for Linda—that allowing her to cry and beg wasn't doing *her* any good, either. But when I suggested to the Fosters that Linda's crying might be a conscious ploy to gain an advantage over them, they seemed surprised, as if they'd never considered the possibility before.

 The more I worked with Linda, the more obvious her learning disabilities became—although differentiating between what Linda couldn't and wouldn't do wasn't always easy.

It was then I decided to try some role-playing. I waited a half hour, until Linda'd calmed down, and then asked another nurse to stay with her for a while. Then, I took the Fosters into an empty room and introduced them to role-playing.

At first, they were shy and embarrassed. I don't think they were accustomed to expressing their feelings—especially in front of a comparative stranger. But then they got into the game. I showed them how their usual responses—guilt, overindulgence, indecision—allowed Linda to take advantage of them, and we practiced some new, firmer responses. I also suggested that when Linda gave them the silent treatment, they try to respond in a more mature way, not by threatening to leave.

"Now why don't you go back in Linda's room and say good-bye—and *mean* it," I said.

I wish I could say that the Fosters' second good-bye went without a hitch, but, of course, it didn't. Linda continued to cry and beg, but the Fosters managed to leave when they said they would, although it must've been hard for them.

After their departure, Linda threw another tantrum and wouldn't let me touch her. Almost an hour later, when her sobs had subsided into an occasional hiccup, I sat down to talk with her. I showed her which buttons to push on the tape recorder, and surprisingly, she caught on quickly. When she heard her family's voices, she cried softly, but this time, she let me hold her hand. After a few minutes, she stopped crying, and then she even started to smile and giggle.

During the next few days, Linda was playing her tapes whenever I entered her room. She'd even memorized parts of them. She had only two tapes, but she seemed happy listening to them over and over. Perhaps the predictability and familiarity of the tapes were as comforting to her as the sound of her family's voices.

At her parents' next visit, Linda tried her whole bag of tricks—pouting, the silent treatment, begging, crying. But my 2 weeks of play therapy were starting to pay off, because Linda showed more control when her parents stood up to leave—she cried, not screamed. The Fosters showed more control, too. When Linda begged them not to go, they told her they *had* to. Then they kissed her, said they loved her, and left the room.

This time, Linda let me hold her while she cried. "Let's play your tapes," I said, and after a few minutes she stopped crying and just listened quietly.

Although Linda never seemed happy while she was hospitalized (and who could blame her), she was much more tranquil than before. Her postoperative period went smoothly—she required less pain medication, cried less often, rang her buzzer only occasionally, and wasn't as fearful about injections or dressing changes. Her parents stayed only 1 day after Linda's surgery, and when they left, Linda kept her crying under control. I told her she'd be going home in 3 weeks, and together we counted the days on her calendar.

I think Linda's parents learned something about themselves and about Linda during her stay with us. They learned that guilt is a wasted emotion—it solves nothing. And that Linda, by *losing* control, was actually controlling *them*.

I learned something too—that role-playing is effective for parents *and* children.

Suddenly Blind at 80

BETTY J. REYNOLDS, RN, MSN

A major life crisis can make a person more susceptible to physical illness—according to a popular psychological theory. Mrs. Stone was a perfect, tragic example of this theory. Because 1 year after her husband's death, 80-year-old Mrs. Stone became suddenly, unexplainably blind.

Mrs. Stone's family doctor had hospitalized her immediately and called in an ophthalmologist and a psychiatrist. At first, the doctors suspected conversion-reaction—a hysterical response to her husband's death. But after many sessions with the psychiatrist and several days of tests, they labeled her blindness of "unknown origin." After a week in the hospital, Mrs. Stone was discharged to the long-term care facility where I work.

None of us had ever cared for a newly blind patient—we couldn't even find any literature on the subject. I was assistant director at the facility and hadn't expected to be involved in Mrs. Stone's physical care. But when the director of nursing asked me to be Mrs. Stone's primary care nurse, I welcomed the challenge.

When I studied Mrs. Stone's chart, I saw that except for her blindness, she was healthy for an 80-year-old. I talked to her family doctor, who'd known her for years—both professionally and socially. He told me that Mrs. Stone's husband had been a prominent surgeon and that the Stones had traveled widely and had been enthusiastic concertgoers and theatergoers. Before her blindness, Mrs. Stone had enjoyed reading, sketching, needlework, and gardening. But her first love was writing poetry, and she'd had several of her poems published.

How tragic, I thought, that so many of the things she loved could now exist for her only in memory. I promised myself I'd help Mrs. Stone again enjoy some of the things she loved.

I decided to spend an hour every day just talking with my patient and getting to know her. Not wanting to frighten her, I introduced myself as soon as I stepped through her door.

She was propped up on pillows, her hands nervously twisting a handkerchief. When she heard my voice, she turned in my direction, staring anxiously at me with sightless eyes.

"Would you like to chat a while, Mrs. Stone?" I asked. "Perhaps you'd like to tell me a little about yourself—you've had such an interesting life, your doctor told me."

"Yes, I had a good life, but now. . . ." Her eyes filled with tears. "Losing your husband's terrible, but I was making it back. Now I'm helpless. It's too much to bear."

I wanted to pat her hand and tell her not to worry, that everything would be fine. But everything *wouldn't* be fine, not while she thought of herself as an invalid. I had to get her out of bed and interested in life again. And I had to help her regain her dignity.

Regaining your dignity isn't easy, though, when you can't eat without spilling your food, and you can't use the bathroom without two nurses escorting you there. We encouraged Mrs. Stone to feed herself, but the food always dribbled down her chin onto her bosom. When she realized what she'd done, she'd burst into tears. Then, when *we* fed her, she'd cry again, saying, "I'm worse than a baby."

She worried constantly that she wouldn't make it to the bathroom on time and rang her call bell frantically when she had to use the toilet. The night nurses complained she was "on the bell" all night. She wanted a glass of milk, she needed to use the bathroom. Sometimes, she only wanted another human being in the room to chase away the loneliness.

I asked the night nurses to report problems with Mrs. Stone that happened during their shift. Every morning they told me the same story—she wasn't sleeping, and she seemed lonely. Couldn't we move her closer to the nurses' station so they wouldn't have to run to the end of the hall 15 times a night?

I wanted Mrs. Stone moved, too—because I knew she felt isolated in her corner room. But her daughter had specifically requested a quiet room, thinking her mother would sleep better away from the noise of the nurses' station. And I couldn't convince her that a little noise might *help* her mother sleep, by making her feel less lonely.

Mrs. Stone's daughter spent at least 12 hours a day in her mother's room—combing her hair, giving her manicures, feeding her, and often, just watching her sleep. "Mother can't eat by herself, so I don't know why you're forcing her to try," she'd say, spooning oatmeal into Mrs. Stone's mouth. Being very polite, Mrs. Stone never dis-

couraged her daughter from waiting on her, but she never really encouraged her, either. We weren't sure how Mrs. Stone felt about this role reversal, but the time wasn't right yet to speak directly to Mrs. Stone about it.

Once Mrs. Stone grew to trust me, she began confiding in me. I shared some of my private life with her, and she, in turn, spoke of her youth, her 62-year marriage, and her children. She tearfully admitted she'd expected to live with her daughter, but that her son-in-law had put his foot down. An elderly blind lady would just disrupt his household. Hearing this, I felt even sorrier for Mrs. Stone, but I also felt sorry for her daughter. No wonder the woman literally jumped every time her mother moved—she was burdened by guilt feelings.

But Mrs. Stone needed more than just her daughter—she needed a whole "family" of people she could trust. She'd always been independent, but now, she was forced to lean on us. And each hour we spent with her brought us a little closer to being her "trustable family."

We assigned four special aides to Mrs. Stone, two for the day shift, and two for the evening shift. We held inservice classes so they'd know how to help her relearn her daily activities.

We made instructional cards that detailed the little lessons we were teaching her and posted the cards wherever the activities would occur. So if I, or one of the aides, was away from the unit when, for example, Mrs. Stone's oral care needed to be done, the substitute could follow the routine outlined on the card over the sink. Doing things the same way every time helped Mrs. Stone relearn the simple tasks she'd once taken for granted. She actually seemed to enjoy following the rules, because if a well-meaning visitor wasn't using the correct procedure, she'd always mention the appropriate card and politely suggest that he read it.

After almost 3 months, Mrs. Stone still hadn't attempted to explore her surroundings. Mostly, she sat in a chair, apathetic and withdrawn. She went only where people led her. So the recreational therapist and I modeled her room in miniature from scraps of pressed wood and cardboard.

The first time we put the model into her lap, Mrs. Stone didn't even want to touch it. She was as bewildered as a child with a road map—she couldn't seem to connect the matchbox furniture with the real furniture in her room. But every day she spent some time feeling the position of the model furniture, then pacing off the room with us. Finally, after 9 days, Mrs. Stone's face suddenly lit up when she fingered the toy furniture. Then, slowly, she began to move around the room unassisted, while we stayed close by. To make sure her world remained exactly as she conceptualized it, we posted still more signs in her room—warning visitors, cleaning persons, and staff members not to *dare* move a stick of furniture.

With our help, Mrs. Stone was finally showing an interest in her surroundings and seemed to accept us as a trustworthy family. Now, we decided, was the time to call in a *real* expert—a person trained to teach blind people how to be mobile— a peripatologist.

The peripatologist spent an hour three times a week with Mrs. Stone—right after her afternoon nap, when she was rested and most receptive to learning. His ultimate goal was to give her the confidence to walk in the hall, unassisted, using handrails or a walker. But 6 months would pass before she'd achieve this goal.

The peripatologist also helped me plan a series of inservice workshops on caring for blind patients. The first workshop, for nurses and aides, taught us how to help a blind person ambulate.

The second workshop, on eating methods for the blind, was for dietitians and kitchen staff, maids, and nursing staff. We blindfolded ourselves and practiced cutting meat, loading forks, and pouring and drinking fluids. Everyone worked in pairs, first feeding themselves and then being fed by a partner. After that, plate guards were never forgotten, and food was always precisely placed on the plate: potatoes at 2 o'clock, meat at 6 o'clock, vegetables at 10 o'clock. Dishes and silverware were put where they belonged on the trays. We never again fed too fast or stuffed food into waiting mouths without announcing what we were presenting.

We also held an inservice workshop to show how a blind person feels when he's approached without explanation. We posted a sign on Mrs. Stone's door asking all visitors to knock and announce themselves. The staff learned the lesson well, but some of the other patients didn't get the message.

One patient, an 85-year-old Italian widower, roamed the halls constantly, talking to himself in half-Italian, half-English. One day he wandered into Mrs. Stone's room, and when she asked, "Who's there?" he didn't answer. He frightened her badly.

We told Mrs. Stone about the patient—how lost he was since his wife's death, and how he refused to eat because he was so grief stricken. Could she think of any way we might help him?

"Perhaps he'd eat if he had someone to eat with," she suggested.

This was the first time Mrs. Stone had reached out to help another person. Up to this point, she'd been totally self-absorbed. Encouraged, we set up a table in her room, and Mrs. Stone and the other patient began eating together. Communicating with a man who spoke broken English wasn't easy for Mrs. Stone, but she tried very hard, and soon, they became good friends.

After a few days, Mrs. Stone went to the patients' dining room for the first time since her admission—accompanied by her friend. With a companion who needed *her* support, she was able to overcome her own embarrassment about her awkward eating skills.

Once she began eating in the dining room and got to know some of the other patients, her self-confidence grew. She began happily awaiting the next activity of the day. We gave her a clock with the crystal removed so she could tell time with her fingers. Each day of accomplishment was followed by a new challenge.

After 9 months, she could find her way around her room without our help, and she learned at last to use the toilet without assistance. She could also step in and out of the bathtub with only one nurse helping her and could bathe herself. We ordered talking books and recordings of her favorite operas and plays, and she listened to them for hours. One day she remarked, "There's so much to be learned!" and we knew she'd taken a big step toward independence.

But every time we hinted gently that we wished she'd write some poetry, she shook her head and said, "I'm not ready for that." Nevertheless, she was willing to learn to use a writing tool.

We cut quarter-inch (0.6-cm) horizontal slots in an 84x11-inch (21.3x27.5-cm) piece of cardboard, placed the cardboard over a sheet of paper, and attached them to a clipboard. Using her left index finger as a guide, she learned to move her pen along the slots. First, she practiced writing letters of the alphabet, then she progressed to words. One day, she told us she didn't need our help to write anymore; that she'd prefer to be left alone. When we visited her an hour later, she proudly showed us a letter she'd written—a simple, loving note to her son in Florida.

We were greatly encouraged by Mrs. Stone's progress, but some problems were still unresolved. For instance, her daughter's almost constant presence. Even though her daughter knew her mother was becoming more and more independent, she still insisted on trying to do everything for her. Every time she said, "Here mother, let me feed you so you won't get your dress all dirty," we cringed. Mrs. Stone seemed torn between wanting to be independent again and letting her daughter "do" for her. Finally, we called a conference and asked her daughter to attend. She listened as staff members, the psychiatric social worker, the chaplain, the peripatologist, and the facility's administrator tried as tactfully as possible to suggest she visit less frequently. At first, she looked angry and hurt, but then she admitted she was exhausted by her constant bedside vigil. Her husband and children were feeling neglected, too, she said.

Still, she resisted our advice for another 2 weeks before she finally began limiting her visits to 3 hours a day. Not surprisingly, Mrs. Stone coped well with her daughter's shortened visits.

The second problem was Mrs. Stone's periods of depression. About once a month, she'd have two or three "down" days, when she lapsed into near silence. We respected her need for privacy and could certainly understand why she might feel depressed sometimes. Actually, we felt it was nothing short of a miracle that she wasn't depressed more often. When she stopped talking, we'd let it ride for a few days and wouldn't press her. But if the depression persisted, I'd try to lead her out of it by asking an open-ended question.

"The last time you and I really talked was Sun-

day," I'd gently remind her. "Today's Tuesday, and I know your mind's been moving along. I wonder. . . ." Usually, Mrs. Stone didn't allow the sentence to dangle—she'd pick up where I left off and tell me what was bothering her. But occasionally, I'd have to make her a bit angry before I'd get a response. "When your children were small, what was the thing they'd do to make you most angry?" I'd say. Thinking back that way would always get her mind active again.

As the months passed, Mrs. Stone talked more about her husband, remembering the good years they'd had together. She spoke optimistically about her future and all the things she still wanted to learn. We felt she'd at last accepted her husband's death. And, just as important, she seemed to accept the fact that she'd probably spend the rest of her life at our facility.

We decided that after 62 years of an unusually close relationship with her husband, Mrs. Stone would appreciate a man's companionship—especially if the man had similar interests and similar problems. We asked for help from the state association for the blind, and they sent us Jabe, an elderly man who lived on his own, although legally blind. Jabe visited Mrs. Stone several times a week, and we'd often hear them discussing books and plays or listening to operas.

Mrs. Stone had been our patient for over a year, and we'd seen her change from a dependent, timid invalid back into the independent, capable woman she'd always been. One warm, April morning, we took her out on the porch—her first trip outside since her admission. We told her the trees were just beginning to bud and the daffodils were blooming. She said, "The breeze feels so warm, and I can smell the earth." We sat on the porch for a long time, and when she returned to her room, she asked for her writing tool. "Tomorrow, I'll have a surprise for you," she said.

The next morning, Mrs. Stone proudly handed us her surprise—the first poem she'd written in over a year. It glowingly described a spring day, *felt* but not seen.

We knew then, she'd made it back.

Ron Taught Us to Expect the Unexpected

LISA MATIAK-MOZINGO, RN, BSN

Helping your patient overcome his fear and anxiety is all in a day's work for most nurses. But our patient, Ron Dorin, turned the tables on us. His obsessive-compulsive behavior was so baffling, *we* became as fearful and anxious as he was.

Thirty-four-year-old Ron had apparently fallen asleep at the wheel before his sports car struck a tree. When he arrived in our orthopedic unit at 8:30 one night, he was a grim sight—I.V.s; nasogastric tube; wired jaw; arm and leg casts; lacerations and contusions; and a skull fracture. For the rest of the shift, we fought to keep him alive. If we could get him through those first few critical hours, we felt he'd make it.

And he did. When I returned to work the next evening, Ron was very much alive and even rewarded me with a weak smile. I decided to tell him then about the ways he could participate in his care, and how this would hasten his recovery.

I explained that by coughing he could bring viscous secretions in front of his jaw wires, so we could suction him more effectively. He coughed right away. I also told him that when he felt stronger, he could give himself partial sponge baths every morning.

"Anything I can do to help—anything that'll make me well faster, just let me know," he said. "And please, call me Ron."

Ron was so cooperative and friendly, I wanted to know more about him. A few days after his admission, I asked my head nurse for permission to look at his complete chart in our medical records department. His chart said he was a lawyer and had an athletic background—team sports, regular exercise, weight lifting. Being in top physical condition before his accident had probably saved his life.

But I wasn't prepared for the next form—it was from a local mental hospital. Two years before, Ron had been hospitalized for a psychotic break, probably caused by his inability to cope with stress. His diagnosis: obsessive-compulsive type, possible paranoid schizophrenia. Reading this, I felt my composure begin to waver. *He certainly seems normal enough,* I thought, promising myself then and there that what I'd read wouldn't color my attitude toward Ron or jeopardize our growing rapport.

In spite of my promise to myself, I felt uneasy.

Although Ron continued to be friendly and helpful, I always had in the back of my mind that he might do something bizarre. But he didn't. Instead, he progressed steadily, gaining weight on his diet of eggnog, milkshakes, and bouillon. Tests confirmed no brain damage from his skull fracture.

He'd adjusted remarkably well to hospital life and talked optimistically about his discharge. So, why did I still feel uneasy?

Then, one morning I gave Ron his bathwater and asked if he'd like to begin his sponge bath. "No," he said, looking surprised and hurt. "I can't."

"But *yesterday* you could," I said, feeling surprised and hurt myself. I patted him on the shoulder and said, "Of course you can, Ron," and went to see my other patients.

When I returned 20 minutes later, the bath tray was still untouched. So, I tried a different suggestion—how would he like to do his mouth care with the water massage? But when Ron tasted the mouthwash, he grimaced in disgust.

"Lisa, you mixed this differently today," he said accusingly. "And it's in the wrong order, too. It's bath, then hair, and *then* mouth. And in an hour, you'll need to change my sheets. And be sure to put a cotton blanket under the bottom sheet to soak up perspiration."

I couldn't believe what I was hearing. Who did he think put the cotton blanket there in the first place? Trying to be calm, I explained that he had to be more independent. Getting no response, I left his room, telling him I'd be back after I saw my *critically ill* patients.

A few minutes later, Ron's call bell buzzed. When I got to his room, he pointed to his I.V. "It burns and it's never done that before. I'll bet you've let it infiltrate."

Now, where did he learn that? I wondered. I checked his I.V., and it was fine. Since he seemed to know all about I.V.s, I told him, "The surrounding tissue is warm, and the I.V. has an excellent blood return." Then, knowing I must've sounded short-tempered, I assured him we'd keep a close eye on his I.V.

"And don't let it run dry, either," he snapped. "Now, while you're at it, I need the urinal." I handed him the urinal and made a fast exit.

"What's wrong with Ron?" I asked the first nurse I saw. She said he'd been giving her problems, too, as well as the other nurses. When I asked what she thought about his surprising amount of medical knowledge, she said, "Didn't you know? He specializes in malpractice cases."

I dreaded going to work the next morning. Ron had definitely turned into a different person—demanding, obsessed with the minutest details of his care. I took a deep breath, opened the door to his room, and was hit with a blast of cold air.

The air conditioner hummed softly, and the blinds were partly drawn. Ron sat in semidarkness, restlessly moving his hands over the bedclothes, as if smoothing out wrinkles. When I turned off the air conditioner and opened the blinds, Ron snapped, "I want that air conditioner on, and the blinds have to be exactly three-quarters closed."

Then he abruptly changed his tone. "Lisa," he said gently, "I know I'm probably not popular with the other nurses, but I know I can ask you for things. Could you please fix my bed? The top has to be 5 inches from the wall, and the left side has to be 1 inch from the nightstand." Confused, I moved his bed the way he wanted it, but I had the distinct feeling I was being manipulated.

During the next few days, Ron's behavior became more and more bizarre. His bathroom door had to be closed at all times, and his food had to be precisely arranged on his tray—meat at 6 o'clock, potatoes at 10 o'clock, vegetables at 2 o'clock. He checked and rechecked the drawer of his nightstand, making sure it was locked. He washed his hands at the slightest provocation. To be honest, he was driving us up the wall.

We wanted to tell Ron to hire a private duty nurse to attend to all his minute whims, but we held our tempers. We remembered what a cooperative patient he'd been and what an intelligent man he was. We asked him what was troubling him, but he denied having any problems. As far as he was concerned, his behavior was just fine the way it was.

One day, I walked into Ron's room and found him stroking a stuffed teddy bear. *Ye Gods, what next?* When he saw my shocked expression, he said petulantly, "I was going to let you pet him, but I've changed my mind." Ron slept with the bear on his pillow every night. When the bear was accidentally caught inside his pillowcase and thrown into the laundry hamper, Ron actually panicked until we found it and returned it to him.

When we realized we were beginning to avoid Ron's room, we decided to hold a team conference. The day of the conference, I had a few free minutes, so I decided to spend them with Ron. His door was half open, so I knocked softly and walked in. When I saw he had a visitor, I turned to leave. Then I realized with a shock that Ron and his

 Ron's behavior became more and more bizarre. His bathroom door had to be closed at all times, and his food had to be precisely arranged on his tray. He kept checking the drawer of his nightstand, to make sure it was locked. He washed his hands at the slightest provocation.

young, male visitor were kissing and caressing! I fled the room as silently as I'd entered. I felt as if I'd been struck. On top of all his other problems, Ron was a homosexual.

Now, we'd have more to talk about at the conference than how to help Ron cope with his problems. If the rest of the team felt as I did, we'd have to discuss how to cope with *our* problems, too.

The other nurses were incredulous when I told them what I'd seen. They, too, felt embarrassed, shocked, and threatened. As we discussed the situation, though, we realized we couldn't consider Ron's homosexuality a "problem." After all, sexual preference is a personal decision. Ron had obviously made his decision and, since it wasn't

a problem for him, we couldn't let it be a problem for us. We promised ourselves not to let our feelings about homosexuality affect our nursing care.

Then we started discussing the *real* problem—his obsessive-compulsive behavior. Although we all had negative feelings about caring for Ron, we all agreed on one point—Ron's *behavior* bothered us, not Ron himself. Even though his obsessive rituals were making him an impossible patient, we still liked the person behind the rituals.

First, we decided to spend all the time we could with Ron—talking to him not just as nurses, but as concerned friends. For the time being, we'd accept his rituals. They seemed to be his way of coping with the stress of immobilization; his way of keeping some control over his environment. We'd continue to urge Ron to be independent and praise him lavishly for his achievements. To give him something concrete to strive for, we planned to ask his doctor to set a definite date for Ron to be out of bed. And we'd ask for a psychiatric consultation.

Ron's doctor agreed to set a date for Ron to get out of bed. But he balked at the idea of a psychiatrist. As far as the doctor was concerned, Ron didn't need a psychiatrist, he needed a boot in the pants. He strode into Ron's room, loomed over his bed, and said, "I want you to throw that damned stuffed animal away and start acting like a man. And I want you out of bed and in a chair tomorrow."

Ron looked wounded to the soul, and I felt terrible. But the next day, the teddy bear was banished to his suitcase, and Ron was out of bed. I can't say I agreed with the doctor's tactics, but they worked.

Getting Ron out of bed was a big step in the right direction, and we followed through on the rest of our care plan right away. We ignored Ron's rituals and concentrated on getting to know him better. We knew he had a strong desire to get well, and we praised him at every opportunity. When we complimented him on his fitness, he literally grinned from ear to ear.

Once Ron was up and around, physical therapy became the high point of his day. He began to set daily goals for himself—walking to the water fountain and back, sitting in the lounge for 15 minutes. We even borrowed a set of barbells so he could exercise in his room. What a joy it was to find Ron lifting weights instead of petting a teddy bear.

Although Ron still retained some of his obsessive rituals, like repeatedly checking his nightstand and washing his hands, he wasn't as rigid about performing them. For instance, he washed his hands *before* meals, but had stopped jumping up to wash them *during* meals. The teddy bear still worried us, though. The toy was out of our sight, but it wasn't out of our minds—and probably not out of Ron's mind, either. We again urged the doctor to order a psychiatric consultation, and he finally agreed.

After talking to Ron, the psychiatrist told us he approved wholeheartedly of our care plan. Continue to ignore the rituals while Ron's performing them, he said. Talk to him about them later.

One day, I was in Ron's room when his dinner tray arrived. I watched him carefully arrange his food, but I just made casual conversation until he'd finished eating. Then I said gently, "Ron, you seem so tense. Can I help?" He finally confided in me. "I just can't stand being stuck in this bed with nothing to do."

Then I had an idea. How would he like to help one of our other patients do her exercises? At first, he was dubious. But when I told him about the 13-year-old girl scheduled for a total hip replacement, who really needed his help to get through her painful exercises, he agreed immediately. "You're really a good person, Ron," I said sincerely. He blushed and said he was glad to help.

Ron had been with us nearly 2 months, and he was almost ready for discharge. We couldn't have been more pleased with his physical progress. We knew he still had some psychological problems to work out, and he'd told us he planned to continue seeing the psychiatrist. All in all, we felt good about Ron and about ourselves.

Ron was discharged after 2 months in our unit. He was going on a vacation with a friend and then planned to return to his law practice, he said. Except for a slight limp, he looked as fit as an athlete.

Caring for Ron was an education for all of us. He taught us to expect the unexpected—and to be ready to meet the challenge. He made us face up to our shortcomings and prejudices—things about ourselves we'd have preferred to ignore. But most of all, he reminded us that every patient has his own way of coping with the stress of immobilization. Ron was certainly an extreme example. But sometimes we need a patient like Ron to make the lesson hit home.

Mrs. Elliot Wasn't Just Overbearing... She Was Overwhelming

REGINA M. MUELLER, RN

The stress of hospitalization can bring out the worst in even the best-tempered person. And if the person wasn't good tempered to begin with, becoming a patient won't improve her disposition. Mrs. Elliot was a perfect example of a difficult person turned difficult patient.

A wealthy, childless widow, the impeccably groomed Mrs. Elliot looked a good deal younger than her 64 years. When she swept off the elevator, her first words to us—delivered rather grandly— were, "I'll have a private room. And here," she took off two diamond rings and a diamond wristwatch, "lock these in the safe."

That scene might have been appropriate in some grand hotel—but in a hospital? What was Mrs. Elliot telling us? That she expected the kind of service from us that she'd get in a luxury hotel? We were soon to find out.

Mrs. Elliot told us she was in the hospital to "have a growth removed." Her growth was actually a malignant tumor of the colon, and she was scheduled for a colon resection in 2 days. Her doctor had decided not to tell her the tumor was cancerous, fearing that if she heard the word "can-

cer," she might give up hope.

Although Mrs. Elliot's manner was, in a word, overbearing, she did cooperate during nursing procedures and tests. That was a relief. Still, she wasn't the kind of patient a nurse could warm up to. The only staff members she seemed to like were the doctors—she called them the "boys" and always combed her hair and put on makeup before they visited her.

Mrs. Elliot tolerated the surgery well, and since the doctors were able to remove the entire tumor, her prognosis was good. We expected she'd be on her way home in 3 weeks.

Frankly, we began counting the days. Because somewhere between the operating room and her return to bed, Mrs. Elliot had changed from an overbearing patient to an overwhelming one.

I was the first to experience the change. The morning after her surgery, when I asked if she'd like to give herself a sponge bath, she snapped, "No, get out of here, you poor excuse for a nurse." I was shocked. What had I done to deserve that?

As the day wore on, Mrs. Elliot increased her demands. We'd run into her room to answer the call light, and she'd point one long, elegant fingernail at the floor and snap, "Pick up that tissue I dropped." And each demand got more petty than the last. "Wipe that spot off my glasses." "Count how many drinking straws I have left." "See if my phone has a dial tone." We all resented being treated like personal servants, but Mrs. Elliot was a sick woman, and we held our tongues.

The next morning, when I saw the angry flash of her call light, I thought, *What now? Does her elastic stocking have a wrinkle?* My first impulse was to ignore the light, but, as it turned out, I *couldn't* ignore it. Even after I pushed the button, the light stayed on.

When I got to her room, I couldn't believe my eyes. In a rage, Mrs. Elliot was tearing her bed padding to shreds and throwing the pieces all over the room. And she'd cleverly pulled the call light out of its socket so it flashed constantly. I sagged wearily against the door. I could hardly believe that this was the same proud, rather grand woman who'd walked off the elevator only 4 days before.

If there was ever a time to write a formal care plan for Mrs. Elliot, this was it. So we held a team conference. We decided that Mrs. Elliot's incessant demands were more than just a bid for attention, that perhaps she was testing us to see if she could trust us to come if she ever *really* needed us.

We decided that to give Mrs. Elliot the best care, we'd have to *share* her care. Every day one of us would take a turn doing her morning care, and we'd see our other patients first, so she'd have our undivided attention. We'd explain our care plan to her so she wouldn't think we were just leaving the worst till last. We'd try to increase her independence by encouraging her to take part in her care. We'd set a few limits for her—for example, she *must* sit in a chair for 20 minutes a day. And, for the time being, we'd simply go along with her other demands, hoping that if she saw how willing we were, she'd settle down.

Well, you know what they say about the best-laid plans. The following day, when I went to do Mrs. Elliot's morning care, I noticed abnormal drainage in her abdominal area. She'd developed a cutaneous fecal fistula. We felt sorry for Mrs. Elliot—the fistula would surely be a terrible blow to her pride. But we also felt sorry for ourselves. Solving her physical problems was our first prior-

ity, and for the time being, the only part of our plan we'd be able to put into effect was sharing her care. And there'd be a lot more care to share, now.

We knew Mrs. Elliot was concerned about her appearance, so we were meticulous about her dressing changes. We put a karaya ring around the fistula, attached a colostomy bag to the ring, and then put 4x4s around the ring to absorb the leakage

 One day, after I'd spent 2 hours caring for Mrs. Elliot, she snapped, "You don't know what you're doing." Her words cut through me like a knife. How could she be so cruel when we were trying so hard?

and keep it from soaking her bedding. We put deodorizers around her room and encouraged her to use her perfumes and powders, to keep the room from absorbing the odor of fecal drainage. To prevent decubiti, we put a foam mattress on her bed and turned her frequently. But every time we turned her on her side, the fistula leaked all over the bed. We had to change her drawsheet and padding every hour.

Mrs. Elliot complained bitterly during the entire turning and dressing change procedure, telling us we were making her worse, not better. One day, after I'd spent 2 hours caring for Mrs. Elliot, she snapped, "You don't know what you're doing." Her words cut through me like a knife. How could she be so cruel when we were trying so hard?

Mrs. Elliot's physical problems didn't improve. Everything she drank drained out of the fistula, and her weight dropped rapidly. The doctors tried intravenous feedings, but her weight continued to drop. So they switched her to total parenteral nutrition (TPN).

After 2 weeks on TPN, Mrs. Elliot was gaining weight, and her physical condition was improving. It was time to start our care plan. We kept our fingers crossed.

I was assigned to Mrs. Elliot the first day of the care plan. I told her that she must sit in a chair for 20 minutes every day. I helped her into the chair, and she grumbled, but at least she didn't scream. As I turned to leave, she was already eyeing the call light. Then I had an idea. "Here's my wristwatch, Mrs. Elliot. You can keep track of the time, too." She took the watch without saying a word, but I could see the relief on her face.

The first few days, Mrs. Elliot tested us by pushing the call light every few minutes. We always responded. Then, miraculously, her calls came less often, until, by the end of the week, she was sitting quietly in the chair for a full 20 minutes. We gradually increased her time, lavishing praise on her if she sat in the chair a few extra minutes.

Because she was feeling better, she began taking pride in her appearance again—she even gave herself partial sponge baths. "Your color's much better," we'd say. "I'm a mess, I'll never get another husband looking like this," she'd grumble. But we could tell she was actually pleased.

We felt that Mrs. Elliot was finally beginning to trust us. During the last 2 weeks, we'd spent so much time caring for her fistula, turning her, and trying to make her comfortable, that she must've realized we *did* care about her. Although she still pushed her call light more than any of our other patients, she didn't make as many meaningless demands. We felt she was calling for us because she was lonely. Sadly, she'd managed to alienate most of her friends because of her constant bickering, so she had few visitors. And since her room was at the end of the hall, she was even isolated from us.

We wondered how Mrs. Elliot would feel about moving to a semiprivate room—she'd been so adamant about a private room when she'd been admitted. We asked her doctor, and he agreed she needed more human companionship. As it was, her only companion was her TV set. So we casually suggested the idea to Mrs. Elliot. At first she didn't respond, but a week later, she told us she'd like a roommate. In 2 hours, she was settled in her new room, just a few steps from the nurses' station.

Moving Mrs. Elliot to a semiprivate room was the best move *we* ever made. And without even planning it, we'd found her the perfect roommate—Mrs. Stevens, who was just as overbearing in her own way. The two women bickered constantly—they couldn't even agree on what TV program to watch. Unlike us, Mrs. Stevens refused to take orders from Mrs. Elliot. But strangely enough, the two women seemed to thrive on the relationship, and Mrs. Elliot never asked to return to her private room.

After 4 weeks of TPN feedings, when Mrs. Elliot had gained 15 pounds (6.8 kg), the doctors decided to close the fistula surgically. "Anything to get out of here," Mrs. Elliot said.

She was anxious to get the surgery over with, and we were anxious, too—for another reason. What kind of mood would she be in *this* time when she returned from surgery?

After her second operation, Mrs. Elliot again changed overnight. I walked into her room, half-expecting to see her tearing her bed padding into shreds. Instead, she greeted me with a big smile. "It's about time you showed up, Regina," she said, but there wasn't a hint of the old sarcasm in her voice. What's more, she'd called me "Regina" instead of "hey you" for the first time since her admission.

What a pleasure it was to see Mrs. Elliot's health and disposition improve. She began drinking clear liquids again, and then, for the first time in weeks, she ate solid foods. The fistula didn't recur.

Mrs. Elliot returned home after 3 months on our unit. When she left, she was still on the thin side, and her face was somewhat pale and drawn, but she was, as always, impeccably groomed. And she swept onto the elevator with the same proud flourish as when she'd arrived.

Looking back, I realize we *did* indulge Mrs. Elliot's whims. But I'm convinced that if we hadn't, she would've remained distrustful and impossibly demanding until the day she left.

And we learned another lesson from caring for Mrs. Elliot. Sometimes nurses have to forget about their pride to help a patient regain hers.

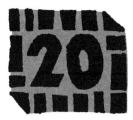

Mr. Gomez Had a Bad Case of "Hospital Smarts"

MARY JO TIERNEY, RN, MS   **DAWN A. TANIGUCHI**, RN, BSN
MARGARET WATSON, RN   **SUSAN I. MAZIQUE**, RN, MPA
JUDITH BETZOLD, RN, BS

Usually, the more familiar a patient is with hospital routines, the better. Not so with Julio Gomez. He knew the hospital ropes so well he could tie us in knots.

As a teenager, Mr. Gomez had both legs amputated in an automobile accident. Since then, recurring sacral pressure sores, diabetic complications, and phantom limb pain had brought him back to our medical/surgical unit many times. Those frequent stays taught him everything he needed to stretch rules, harass staff, and unsettle administrators.

Mr. Gomez, for example, began one stay on our unit by theatrically slapping issues of *The American Bar Review* and *Lawyer* on his windowsill—where no one could miss them. Next he propped various pages from our procedure manual on his bedside stand. Then and only then did he allow us to transfer him from wheelchair to bed. The last thing he said as we left was, "Put the phone here. I'm gonna need it."

Once the stage was properly set, "Mr. Hospital Savvy" went into action.

"This is Mary Ann from admissions. Mr. Gomez in Room 450 just called. He says he wants a new room because the patient across the hall is too noisy."

"Medical records calling. Mr. Gomez in Room 450 wants copies of his current chart. Does he have his doctor's approval on that?"

"Mrs. Jones from hospital administration. Mr. Gomez in Room 450 says his nurses didn't follow the procedure manual when they changed his dressing. Please look into this and call me back."

Mr. Gomez used the phone beyond AT&T's fondest dreams, but he wasn't reluctant to complain in person, either: "You call yourself a nurse, with that sloppy technique? Take a look at this procedure manual—is this the first time you've seen it?"

If he wasn't spreading blame, he was stirring trouble: "You could learn something from the nurse who just took care of me. *She* knows how to make a patient comfortable."

The staff left Mr. Gomez's room with one of two expressions—frustration or relief.

Mr. Gomez was the typical manipulative patient, but in all fairness, he was also using his hospital savvy to protect himself against hospital bureaucracy. After all, who knows the flaws in the system better than the frequent patient?

Problem: Rooms are allocated randomly. Defense: Insist—loudly—on the room you want. Problem: Mistakes can be made in transcribing orders. Defense: Double-, even triple-check medications, procedures, and diets. Problem: Patients are sometimes assigned float nurses unfamiliar with their care. Defense: Demand a particular nurse.

A patient's familiarity with hospital routine can even help his nurses—for example, when he refrains from requesting medication at the change of shift or when he clusters requests to save us unnecessary trips into his room.

But Mr. Gomez had turned his defense into an offense. Instead of giving us a chance to solve problems, he took his complaints straight to the administrators. And why not? Concerned about lawsuits, they usually asked us to placate him. Gradually, our annoyance at Mr. Gomez's manipulations turned into anger. Why should one patient be allowed to take up so much of our time? What about patients who needed more care than Mr. Gomez—who spoke up for them? Why should administrators listen to a patient when he hadn't even tried talking to us?

Mr. Gomez was being unfair to us and, ironically, to himself. By going over our heads, he deprived himself of the help we could have supplied to keep him out of the hospital. For instance, he ignored our advice about preventing skin problems through proper body positioning, exercise, and good nutrition. Nor would he accept our offers to teach him biofeedback, relaxation, hypnosis, or other pain control techniques.

Things came to a head the morning of Mr. Gomez's discharge. He had asked the nursing office, social service, *and* an ambulance company to arrange transportation home. Luckily, our unit head nurse discovered this before three drivers arrived to pick him up.

So when Mr. Gomez called a month or two later to find out when his favorite room (you guessed it, Room 450) would be available, we knew his next move would be to call his doctor to have himself admitted. This time, we prepared.

Our head nurse called a conference, inviting the director of nursing, Mr. Gomez's doctor, and representatives from various departments. We discussed how we'd inadvertently reinforced Mr. Gomez's demanding behavior with visits from supervisors, calls from other departments, and assignment of nurses he requested. One of those

Gradually, our annoyance at Mr. Gomez's manipulations turned into anger. Why should one patient be allowed to take up so much of our time?

nurses, Juana, said, "Being admitted to a hospital always means losing some control over your life, but this may be even more of a threat to Mr. Gomez because of his disability. In his personal life, he can avoid situations that draw attention to it—he goes only to restaurants that can easily accommodate him, and so on. And since his home is designed around his wheelchair, he's very much in control—there. Here, he's dependent on us.

"Maybe this loss of control brings back the grief reaction he felt 20 years ago," she continued. "He may be remembering how he felt at first: perhaps, 'If I can't walk, I'm no longer a man... I won't live like this.'"

"Hospitalization may also remind him of another source of tension in his life—his racial minority status," Ann added. "Any situation that restricts his freedom may seem threatening: 'You'd better fight for yourself...no one else will...let the world know you're not someone to be messed with.'"

"We can't forget the role medication plays, either," said Mary. "Mr. Gomez takes large doses of analgesics at home for phantom limb pain, but we reduce the dosage here—and withdrawal might contribute to his edginess and erratic behavior.

"Understanding why he wants control is only part of the solution, of course. Now, what can we do to change the behavior?"

That's when we all took a look at the system Mr. Gomez knew so well. Could we improve it? For instance, wouldn't insisting on a first-come, first-served basis for allocating beds be fairer? And what about patient assignments? Should Mr. Gomez be able to pick and choose his nurses? The director of nursing suggested that, instead, Mr. Gomez be assigned a primary nurse. This would ensure consistency of care for him.

And could we find a way to stop Mr. Gomez from enlisting several departments to handle a single problem (and give his dialing finger a rest)? The director of nursing promised to refer Mr. Gomez back to the unit, and she asked other department heads to do the same. As a reminder, we distributed a synopsis of our conference to our nursing staff and the other employees Mr. Gomez called frequently.

A few days later, Mr. Gomez again swept into Room 450, snapped open a briefcase, and propped *The Manual of the Joint Commission on Accreditation of Hospitals* against his water pitcher. (Give the man credit: He *was* resourceful.)

This time we were prepared. Within minutes his primary nurse, Mary, introduced herself to him. Within an hour they'd formulated a written contract summarizing his expectations of his nurses as well as their expectations of him. Included in this was a schedule of events for the day so Mr. Gomez would know what would happen next.

Mary also won Mr. Gomez's trust by visiting him often "just to talk." Eventually, some of his feelings about his hospitalization emerged. "You know," he said, "Twenty years ago, just 2 months after my wedding, I was on my way to pick up my wife when a tractor-trailer hit me. The next thing I was in a hospital—with my legs gone. God, you have to be on your guard all the time."

Taking his hand, Mary said, "I'm sure the doctors who performed your surgery were working in your best interests, Mr. Gomez. But I agree, watching out for your rights is important. You can relax a little now—I'm watching out for you, too." She then asked him to keep a list of any problems he encountered, including the time and date. She'd add the intervention.

Here's an example. Problem: Didn't get what I wanted on my dinner tray, 6 p.m., 4/12. Intervention: RN called dietitian, 4/13.

Only if the two of them couldn't resolve a problem would the director of nursing intercede, and she'd always call Mary in whenever she talked to Mr. Gomez. This way, all "sides" were represented. Afterward, Mary would chart their solutions in the nurses' notes or care plan so everyone would be aware of them.

Because our care plans became more specific, our care became more consistent—and Mr. Gomez couldn't play us against each other. To foster that continuity, we urged float nurses to discuss the care plans with us before they met him.

Moreover, if a problem on the list had legal implications, Mary discussed it with the quality assurance department. And as agreed during the conference, whenever Mr. Gomez called administration or other departments, he was directed back to Mary, with a polite, "We're concerned about your care, Mr. Gomez, but please ask your primary nurse to call us after you've discussed this with her." No more headaches created by too many people working on the same problem.

Did this mean Mr. Gomez became a docile patient? Hardly—but that wasn't our primary goal. What we wanted was to switch his focus from manipulating the system to improving his health.

It seemed to work. Once he was spending less time complaining on the phone, he spent more time listening to our patient teaching. He slowly seemed to realize that his old tactics wouldn't get him anywhere, but following our self-care instructions might just get him home—to stay.

On the day of his discharge, Mr. Gomez gave us subtle proof of his changed attitude. He was carefully packing the patient-teaching booklets we'd given him into his briefcase when he paused, obviously struggling with some decision. Sighing, he said, "Guess I won't have room for this," then took out his JCAH manual and slid in a nutrition handbook.

It felt good to think that Mr. Hospital Savvy had finally "wised up."

Battle Cry for Mr. MacDonald

JULIE D. MALCOLM, RN, BSN

We sometimes forget that the person we treat in the hospital or nursing home is, in a sense, two people—one, the sick, dependent patient we actually see; the other, the person he is in the outside world. Our problem in treating Mr. MacDonald, a 74-year-old resident of the nursing home where I work part time, was that we focused only on the *patient*.

Mr. MacDonald had been a top executive and key labor negotiator for a large manufacturing firm. He had suffered a cerebrovascular accident, resulting in hemiparesis on the left side. Wheelchair-bound, he could walk only with assistance and had become so dependent in just about every way that his wife couldn't care for him at home. A distinguished-looking, heavyset man, he was also on a 1,200-calorie, low-sodium diet because of high blood pressure and his weight problem.

Mr. MacDonald, who spoke with a slight Scottish brogue, was a complex, brilliant man. On the one hand, he was a social leader for the other residents—he led a Bible study group and occasionally gave slide presentations about his extensive travels. On the other hand, he was a problem

for the staff—he wouldn't cooperate with his treatment and used many ploys to manipulate us—and, indeed, wear us out. I fell for one of them, in fact, the very first day I met him.

Soon after a nursing assistant had wheeled him back from the dining room and helped him into bed for a nap, he called to me as I walked past his door. Would I wheel him down the hall, where he had something important to discuss with one of the other residents? Since I was on an errand, I asked if he could wait about 10 minutes.

"Ah," he said wearily, "when I was a wee lad in Scotland, I had to work in the mines. Had the strength of two men, mind you. Now I'm a mistreated, forgotten old man who has to beg for a few minutes down the hall."

Flushed with guilt, I helped him back into the wheelchair. As he settled in, he noted my surname on my name tag. Ah, Scottish, he said—was I familiar with the poems of Robert Burns?

"There's one you call to mind," he said. Then looking at me: "'As fair art thou, my bonnie lass / So deep in love am I / And I will love thee still, my dear / Till all the seas gang dry.'"

What a charmer—I would have pushed his wheelchair halfway across the state. In fact, I wasn't all that upset when I found out he didn't really want to talk to anyone down the hall—he'd either simply wanted to go for a ride or to put me to work. Furthermore, I still thought him charming when I learned from my co-workers that this was one of his techniques for winning favors—he'd joke, flirt, make wisecracks, or quote from scripture and his favorite authors.

However, he could also be unreasonably demanding. Instead of cooperating in his treatment—for instance, trying to learn how to put on some of his clothes—he'd insist, "That's your job!" Not only was he reinforcing his dependency and closing the road to rehabilitation, but he was also depleting his self-esteem by forever referring to himself as a "forgotten old man."

And his refusal to accept responsibility for anything he did was far from charming. For example, one day a nursing assistant found a cache of chocolate-chip cookies in his drawer. When I asked him why he was cheating on his diet, he denied it.

"I just like to have some little sweets around," he said. "They remind me of the days when I didn't have to beg for a bit of kindness."

"You're still not losing any of the weight you should."

"Ah," he said with a wave of disgust, "that's because of the highly caloric food they serve here."

Why didn't he at least go to any of the exercise classes, especially in light of his diminishing range of motion? "They don't have enough classes," he replied, ignoring the fact that he didn't go to *any*. What's more, he said, all his problems would be solved if the staff would just go along with what he wanted. "What we need here is more staffing."

As I started to leave, he suddenly smiled and raised his unaffected arm with a clenched fist. "Scots, wha hae," he said.

When I asked him what the phrase meant, he said it was part of another Robert Burns poem, a sort of rallying call to battle, which roughly meant "All Scots that are here." As he went on to recite the rest of the verses of what actually seemed to be a brutal battle call, I stared at him with a kind of tingling in my spine. To me, this meant that somewhere in him was a stubborn will to fight to the end—if we could only reach it and strengthen it. And I decided to make that my goal.

When I discussed my plans with my co-workers, we agreed that a "battle" was indeed raging in Mr. MacDonald—the current dependent patient versus the former high-powered executive. And the dependent patient obviously was winning. Moreover, the executive in him might be reacting to the care he needed in the way he reacted to past business problems. In other words, he could be delegating responsibility for his care to the staff because he didn't see it as his responsibility.

I sat down with Mr. MacDonald and discussed what I wanted to do in terms an executive could appreciate. I wanted to make a "contract" with him for a treatment plan. According to the contract, he wasn't to try to entertain or divert me during our sessions with such things as quotes or jokes. He was to table them for later. Instead, our sessions would be devoted strictly to discussing his problems and possible solutions.

At this meeting, for the first time, some of his doubts about himself poured out. He, too, was frustrated—indeed, depressed—that his tactics hadn't helped improve his health. But, though he said he doubted that any new approach would work, he would try.

My first goal was to help him raise his self-esteem, to see himself—as many of us did—as the home's most vibrant resident rather than as a woe-heavy old man. I asked him to make a sort of "annual report," to list all of his accomplishments in the home, as well as his long-range plans.

He took to the task enthusiastically and later read off his accomplishments with great satisfaction. These included directing the Bible study group and giving the travel lectures, making calligraphy place cards in the dining room for the residents, and relating well to others. His long-range plans were as elaborate as running a mail-order business for gourmet cooking supplies and hosting a retreat house for Christian travelers in Nova Scotia. His main goal right now, though, was to "get out of this prison and go home."

He admitted, however, that he couldn't go home until he became less dependent. So, we set up an intermediate goal—to be transferred to the west wing, which was for residents who required less care. First, though, he'd have to relearn some basic skills in caring for himself. For instance, he'd have to walk more, lose weight, help us dress him, and be more consistent in maintaining bladder control.

To try to win his cooperation, I appealed to the labor negotiator he'd once been. Because he had a number of complaints about his care, I told him we would "bargain for concessions," a term that struck a spark into this corporate warrior's eyes.

One of his complaints, for example, was that he thought bladder training was demeaning—"I'm not a dog to have to do it on command." He wanted to be trusted to use his urinal consistently. Another complaint was that he didn't want staff insisting that his door be open when he wanted it closed. I agreed that we wouldn't impose any institutional routines on him without first consulting him. On his part, he—besides agreeing to such things as walking more—would stop telling "poor me" stories.

"It's a deal," he said, holding out his hand.

"A deal," I said, shaking it. Then, at the doorway, I turned and looked at him. "Scots, wha hae."

He grinned and clenched his fist.

During the next several weeks, he made small but significant progress—for instance, he used his unaffected arm to help us put on his shirt, walked more, lost a few pounds, and had better control of his bladder. We were able to transfer him to the west wing.

Soon afterward, however, he showed signs of regressing. When I asked him what was the matter, he responded with a quote from Shakespeare. "I'm just," he said, "'a wretched soul, bruised with adversity.'"

"I thought," I said, "we made a contract that you weren't going to say things like that about yourself."

As we talked further, the truth came out—the move to the west wing frightened him.

"I'm afraid everyone's going to expect too much of me here," he said, "I'm afraid I won't be able to keep up."

No one, I assured him, was expecting anything beyond what we were sure he was capable of doing.

"Or is your real reason," I suggested with a smile, "that you're just trying to renegotiate the contract?" His lips formed a little smile, too, and he shook his head.

During the next few weeks he worked hard at being more independent. Sometimes, when things just seemed too much for him, I'd try to encourage him with that rallying cry. And, again, he began making slow but discernible progress—lost a few more pounds (his blood pressure also came down), took more and longer walks, cooperated more with the staff. Then one day I came to work and saw with a plummeting heart that his bed was empty.

A nursing assistant had found him in a coma the night before, and he'd been taken to a hospital. He'd suffered another massive cerebrovascular accident.

I went to see him as soon as I could. His eyes were closed; he was breathing through an oral airway. He seemed to have shrunk beneath the folds of his skin. I walked slowly to his bed and took his hand. I said, "Mr. MacDonald."

No response

"It's me, Mr. MacDonald. Julie Malcolm."

Still nothing.

Then, still holding his hand, and my eyes suddenly filling with tears, I said, "Scots, wha hae."

Instantly a chill ran through me: His eyes opened ever so slightly.

I sat down next to his bed and took his Bible from his night table. I read several of his favorite chapters to him, and finished with one section from Phillipians I knew he especially loved: "In Him who is the source of my strength I have strength for everything."

As I stood up to leave, his eyes remained closed. But his mind, I was sure, was as active as ever. I would, I resolved, keep working with him, even though it surely meant starting from the very beginning. He'd taught me so much—about myself and the care of patients—that he didn't need to raise a clenched fist to rally me to his cause.

"I'm here, Mr. MacDonald. Scots, wha hae."

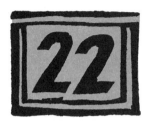

Mr. J.J. Sylvester Was a Real Con Artist

RITA SPILLANE, RN, MSN

For some patients, manipulation is an art form. They'll try anything to avoid doing what you want them to do. And if they're really good at being bad, you won't even know it. That's why I call them the con artists.

As far as I'm concerned, Mr. J.J. Sylvester—*and don't forget the 'J.J.'*—was the Picasso of con artistry. Sixty-seven years old, he suffered from Parkinson's disease, and at 5 feet 4 inches (160 cm) tall, he weighed barely 100 pounds (45 kg). But his mind was sharp and his imagination was rich…at least when it came to disrupting his care plan.

Hindsight, you know. They say it's 100% accurate, but that first day I never would've guessed the tiny shape curled pathetically on the stretcher could cause so many problems. As the two burly ambulance attendants wheeled the stretcher past the nurses' station, all of our heads turned at once. "Help me, help me," a weak voice cried from under the sheet. Concerned, I gave chase.

I arrived at the patient's room just as the attendants were transferring him into bed. "Help me, help me," he called out again, quickly pulling the sheet over his head. When I asked what was happening, one of the attendants rolled his eyes and said, "Nurse, this guy'll drive you bananas if you listen to everything he says."

But I soon learned my patient was in pain—and for some pretty believable reasons. He'd spent the past 3 months in another hospital, where he'd been treated for a bleeding ulcer. While there, he'd developed two decubitus ulcers, one on his buttock and the other on his sacrum. Now, the slightest movement or pressure near those gaping ulcers caused him agony.

But that's not all that brought him to our 200-bed rehabilitation hospital. He had such severe contractures that he lay in a fetal position, knees drawn up to his chin.

As I introduced myself, I watched his fingers manipulate the bedsheet in characteristic pill-rolling tremor. His masklike face and large, staring eyes were clear indications of parkinsonism. Like most victims of that affliction, Mr. Sylvester spoke in a barely audible, monotonous tone, but when he looked at me and said, "Help me," my heart went out to him. "I'll try," I said sincerely.

Following medication orders, I administered 50 mg meperidine (pethidine, Demerol) for pain. Soon afterward, he told me about his experiences in the first hospital. "They tried to kill me," he explained, without blinking. "They were so cruel and terrible, they treated me like a dog. Except I had a dog once, and I treated him better than they treated me."

Sensing he'd hooked me (there were even tears in his eyes), he launched into a tale about the osteomyelitis he'd had as a child. "I was terribly sick, let me tell you," he said, "and I hardly had a friend in the world. You know what it's like to be a boy and not have a friend in the world? And now I have scars all over my legs. Just look... everywhere."

After 20 minutes, I wasn't feeling pity for my patient anymore. By that time, I was feeling pretty distracted and decided to interrupt him. Knowing he was nonambulatory, I asked, "When was the last time you walked, Mr. Sylvester?"

That question did stop him—but not the way I'd anticipated. He glared at me so long and hard I thought he might be looking for some family resemblance.

"What's the matter?" I finally said.

"Don't ever call me that."

"Call you what?"

"Don't you *ever* call me Mr. Sylvester," he said. "My name is Mr. J.J. Sylvester."

"Well, that shouldn't be a problem, J.J.," I said, making a note on his Kardex.

"Not *J.J.*," he growled, even angrier than before. "*Mr. J.J. Sylvester.* Get it?"

Not really. But if that's what he wanted to be called, it was fine with me. As I amended the notation I'd just written, I asked him, "What's the J.J. stand for, anyway?"

"That's for me to know and for you to find out," he answered sharply, pulling the sheet over his head again. I left the room not knowing what to make of my newest patient.

I'd no sooner gotten back to the nurses' station when his call light began glowing. He wanted to talk some more. During the next 3 hours of my shift, his call light lit up exactly 32 times—a unit record. By the end of the day, I was—in the word of the ambulance attendant—bananas.

But later I understood why Mr. J.J. Sylvester

made such a nuisance of himself. He was lonely. His wife had diabetes and hypertension and couldn't visit him often. He seemed to have no other family or friends, and more than anything, he just wanted to go home. Once, he said he was afraid of catching an "affection" and dying. Actually, that's just what I thought he craved—affection.

So we worked out a schedule of staff visitations that kept him occupied during the day. Each nurse encouraged him to talk, and we planned time to spend with him not only teaching but also visiting socially. When we were hurried or he was tired and frustrated, we tried to anticipate his needs, and we asked questions that could be answered with a simple nod of his head.

Our strategy seemed to work. By the third day, his call light lit up only 3 times during my shift.

Of course, we were also giving him decubitus ulcer care every 4 hours, always making sure to medicate him 20 to 30 minutes beforehand to ease his discomfort during the procedure. The dietitian provided high-protein, high-fiber foods, and I encouraged him to drink nutritional supplements such as Sustacal, eggnog, and milk shakes between meals. Because his trembling had made eating increasingly difficult, we had to feed him ourselves, so mealtime became a social occasion, too.

After 2 weeks of improved nutrition, passive range-of-motion (ROM) exercises, and meticulous decubiti care, the ulcers began to granulate and form pink, healthy tissue. Finally, he could move without experiencing searing pain.

Next, after getting him to perform active ROM exercises three times a day, we focused his rehabilitation on activities of daily living. Without that constant exercise, he'd never be capable of sitting, standing, or walking on his own—all prerequisites for returning home. I was very hopeful about his steady progress.

The first sign that things weren't going as smoothly as they seemed was the sudden tension between nursing staff members. What was going on? People who'd cooperated for months—and sometimes for years—were snapping at each other. Staff morale on the unit hit the doldrums, and I couldn't explain it. The first clue that Mr. J.J. Sylvester was the artist behind the discontent came when he casually mentioned to me, "Hey, you know that nurse with short hair…what's her name? She says she doesn't like how you're handling things."

My first response was to talk to the nurse he'd mentioned. From that brief conversation, we quickly surmised that Mr. J.J. Sylvester was spreading divisive rumors about the two of us. Unknown to us at the time, the seeds of disunity were being sown far wider than we guessed.

One day another nurse suddenly stopped me in the hallway to say that what I'd told someone about her "in confidence" was totally untrue. "What are you talking about?" I said incredulously. We both realized then that Mr. J.J. Sylvester was manufacturing more tales.

My first priority, then, was to call a staff meeting to air all the rumors. Afterward we had a good laugh about some of them, and the tension broke. Later that day I gave Mr. J.J. Sylvester a stern talking-to, and he sheepishly agreed to stop passing on rumors he'd "heard." He never admitted starting them.

By the fifth week of rehabilitation, he could sit up for an hour each afternoon. Our next goal was to get him to feed himself. Here, too, his skill at con artistry came into play. After 2 weeks he'd made so little progress eating independently that I figured he was getting help from some of the nurses or, on occasion, his wife. I talked to him about my expectations for making him more independent… which included getting him to feed himself.

"But I'm fading away to nothing," he complained wearily. I knew he wasn't starving, but being aware of his precarious nutritional status, I decided his complaints were certainly worth considering. After all, because of the poor coordination between his hand and mouth he was continually dropping food. Also, he simply refused to eat his food if it was the least bit cold.

During the next few days, we solved these problems. First, we ordered a spoon designed for the handicapped, which can be strapped to the patient's hand. We requested that all of Mr. J.J. Sylvester's meats, vegetables, and fruits be pureed, so less food was lost on the trip to his mouth. At the same time, we offered him plenty of finger foods such as raw vegetables, and we provided straws for easier drinking. We also made sure his

tray was served first and picked up last, so his food was warm and he didn't feel rushed.

To protect his gown and bed, we covered his chest with Chux and always gave him extra napkins. Finally, we tried to leave him alone during mealtimes because no matter how hungry he said he was, he much preferred talking to eating. Mr. J.J. Sylvester finally started feeding himself regularly.

Teaching him how to stand and walk took a lot more effort and patience from us. To motivate him, we capitalized on his strong desire to go to the bathroom rather than use a bedpan, as he'd been doing. His still-tender sacrum made using the bedpan extremely uncomfortable.

First, we established a regular time each day for bowel movements. We'd insert a laxative suppository, then 20 minutes later two of us would assist him to the bathroom. To make him as comfortable as possible, we had a raised toilet seat and handrails installed. Two weeks later, he didn't need the suppositories—he was already right on schedule.

After a month, he progressed from needing the help of two assistants to walk to needing the help of only one. And after another month, he could walk alone with a walker. A few weeks later he began walking with a cane. Like many patients with Parkinson's disease, he had a propulsive gait that made him appear as if he were constantly losing his balance. We taught him to bring his toes up with every step and to spread his legs (10 inches [25 cm]) to provide a wider base for walking and a better stance.

Once he was solidly on his feet, he seemed to enjoy his freedom. When we heard his famous, "Watch out for Mr. J.J. Sylvester," we got out of his way…fast. We knew he'd be coming through.

Now only one task remained for him to accomplish before he could go home: He had to learn to dress himself. To help him as much as possible, we arranged his clothes on the bed while he took his morning bath. Then we left the room and closed the door.

Boy, were we in for a surprise. The first day, he came out of his room fully clothed in less than a half hour. The second day, it took him about 20 minutes to dress. And the third day, he was dressed in 10 minutes flat. His swift progress seemed too good to be true.

Well, it *was* too good to be true. One morning I walked into his room and found Marie, the cleaning woman, helping him on with his clothes.

The moment he saw me, Mr. J.J. Sylvester's face dropped. He knew he'd been caught breaking the rules. Getting caught is the worst possible thing for a con artist. "Marie, I'd like to speak with you, please," I said politely.

Marie parked her mop and bucket outside the nurse's conference room, and we talked. First I explained how important our routine for dressing Mr. J.J. Sylvester was and just how much we needed her cooperation. She looked guilty, then said, "But he seems like such a nice old man who just tells a story or two."

Apparently, he'd complained to her that his nurses were neglecting him. I could hear him now: "Imagine, they won't even help me get dressed." That was how he'd conned her into helping him.

Once Marie understood our plan, though, she stood her ground with Mr. J.J. Sylvester. So he wouldn't be tempted to call her, she cleaned the rooms at the opposite end of the hallway in the morning when he needed her help. The next day, when he couldn't find her, he spent nearly 2 hours getting dressed. But at least he did it all by himself.

Don't relax quite yet. The surprises still weren't over. The following morning, Dr. Lloyd dropped by to visit him. A minute later, he stormed down the hallway toward us. "Why aren't you nurses helping Mr. Sylvester get dressed?" he said. He'd found his patient literally hung up in his tee shirt and trembling all over.

We could only smile at first. Then we explained our plan and told him our patient was capable of dressing himself if given enough time. Suddenly, Dr. Lloyd flushed. "That son of a gun," he chuckled. "He really got me, didn't he?"

Without another word, he returned to Mr. J.J. Sylvester's room, where he emphasized the importance of our step-by-step care plan and instructed his patient to cooperate. "And I thought you were a Christian," Mr. J.J. Sylvester whined as Dr. Lloyd left his room.

Well, cooperate he did—although I think it was a real blow to his ego. What other choice did he have, though? I mean, there was not one nurse, doctor, orderly, or cleaning lady left to con on the entire unit. And our persistence eventually paid off: Just before he was discharged, he could dress himself in 25 minutes. After 4 months in our care, Mr. J.J. Sylvester was ready to live independently at home.

And home, we soon discovered, was probably the only place he'd ever meet his match. On his last day, his wife came to accompany him home. As they left his room, we heard their two voices coming down the hall toward us.

You could hardly tell them apart:

"I'm still in terrible pain."

"Pain? I wish that was the worst of it. The doc tells me my blood pressure's hitting the ceiling."

"You talk about ceilings... I've been staring at the same ceiling day and night for the last 6 months."

"Yeah, but at least you got somebody to care for you."

"Care? You call what I got care? I'm dying."

"Dying? You say you're dying...."

And that was the last time any of us ever saw Mr. J.J. Sylvester. I never learned why he tried to con everyone the way he did. Or why he was so darned good at it. I never learned why he always wanted to be referred to as Mr. J.J. Sylvester. I never even learned what the J.J. stood for.

I'll tell you what I did learn—something valuable about team communication. It means more than just having "nuts and bolts" nursing conferences. Real team communication demands emotional honesty from staff nurses. It means keeping in touch. Nursing patients like Mr. J.J. Sylvester also requires a special cooperation from doctors. And, oh yes, sometimes from the cleaning lady.

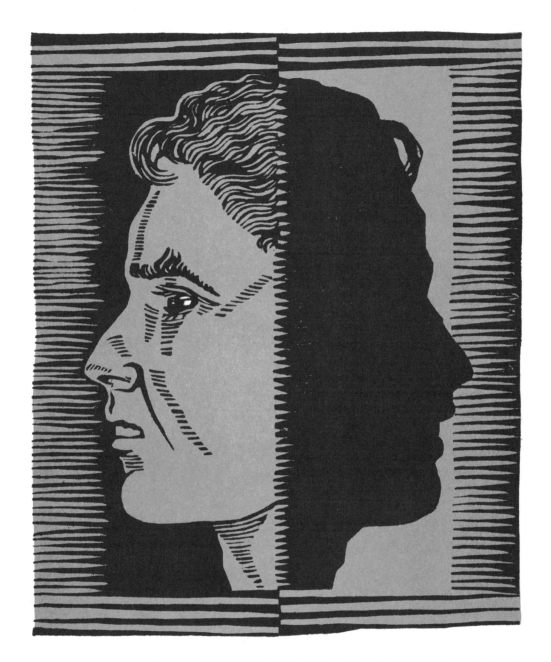

PATIENTS WITH AN ALTERED SELF-IMAGE

In Planning Mr. Bowen's Care, One Picture Was Worth a Thousand Words

COLEEN A. SHOEMAKER, RN, BSN
KAREN SCHAEFER, RN, MSN

Sometimes a patient's condition is so horrendous, so tragic, that we may be tempted to lose ourselves in the technical aspects of his care and try to shut off our feelings. Such a patient was Mr. Bowen, his face as disfigured as anything in a horror movie.

When my head nurse first told me about him, and that I was to be his primary nurse because she thought I could handle the "challenge," I felt my heart contract. His history was a sad one: A 72-year-old bachelor, he'd been a recluse for the past 14 years because of a progressively growing malignancy of the face—which he'd never had treated. The huge tumor had become so gangrenous and foul smelling that his family refused to care for him in his apartment any more. Only then had he finally agreed to undergo surgery.

The surgery—which had lasted 17 hours—involved excision of his midface, including removal of his nose, lips, part of his tongue, and his left eye, then extensive grafting. Later, on a special care unit, he developed an infection in his right eye, which resulted in total loss of vision. He was now being transferred to our general patient unit.

That night, for the first time since I'd been a nurse, I was nervous about meeting a new patient. I kept picturing what he might possibly look like, and each image I conjured up was worse than the next. Still, it didn't prepare me for the sight that awaited me when I walked into his room.

He almost seemed to have no face. The only openings were the empty eye socket; the sightless right eye, which he kept closed; and a small, lipless hole of a mouth.

He lay motionless in an array of tubes—nasogastric, tracheostomy, triple-lumen central venous catheter, and Texas catheter. I felt a surge of pity and—to my dismay—revulsion and actual fear. I was overwhelmed, didn't know if I could indeed handle this challenge.

Mr. Bowen needed so much care I didn't know where to begin. Yet, as his primary nurse, I had to come up with a care plan for all of the shifts. First of all, I wanted to prepare the other nurses for what he looked like. And his needs were so complex that I wanted to set out the details of his care in a way that would make it easier and less stressful for them.

I decided to draw a simple, schematic sketch of

his body, including the various tubes, grafted areas, and donor sites. Then I outlined the daily care plan, referring to the appropriate place on the sketch for each step. The regimen would begin with bathing and skin care. Afterward, we'd apply aloe to all healed graft areas and donor sites. We'd then place gauze soaked in normal saline on his left eye socket and the unhealed graft area on the left side of his chest. Then, after his tube care and decubiti care, we would perform passive range-of-motion exercises, as well as apply knee splints to prevent contractures of his legs.

I felt more in control after devising the care plan, yet I still dreaded going in the next day. I found myself thinking that the only way I could continue caring for Mr. Bowen was to focus all my energy on the procedures, to try not to feel anything. But I dismissed this idea almost at once. I know myself too well. I remember learning as a student how important it is to treat a patient as a person, not an object. I've always become attached to my patients, have always tried to give them emotional support. I couldn't be a nurse any other way.

The next morning, though my heart was rocketing, I managed to say cheerfully, "Good morning, Mr. Bowen. It's me again—Coleen. I don't know if you've lost track of the days but, in case you have, today's Tuesday. And it's a warm, sunny day."

He lay without moving, without even turning his head slightly. He was unable to talk because of the surgery on his tongue. But I knew he could hear.

"They say it's going to be sunny tomorrow, too," I continued, checking his intravenous line and other tubes. "I hope so. We've been having a lot of rain."

I had decided to start off each morning by orienting him to the day and weather and to find things to talk to him about whenever I was in the room. I hoped that hearing the same voice, knowing that at least one person cared for him (he hadn't had a visitor as yet) would make him feel less alone, less cut off from the world. Maybe it would even spark some kind of communication from him.

I became totally comfortable with Mr. Bowen after a few days, though I did feel frustrated by his failure to respond.

In the meantime, of course, we had a host of physical problems to deal with. For instance, though he'd been placed on a fluid-filled bed, his sacral decubitus wasn't healing. I consulted with a burn nurse specialist, who showed me how to debride the dead skin and suggested trying another type of dressing. After about a week we could see signs of healing.

And I got some more help from an unexpected source. Because my sketch and care plan had caught the attention of my head nurse and a clinical nursing instructor at a nearby college, they assigned a student nurse to me. She too always explained procedures to Mr. Bowen and tried, with touching as well as words, to let him know we cared about him.

I also had one of his former nurses from the special care unit visit him in the hope that he would respond to a familiar voice.

"Mr. Bowen"—she leaned toward him—"do you remember me? Sue? I took care of you downstairs?"

He didn't stir.

She said, "If you feel me holding your hand, squeeze my hand. Please."

But nothing. After several more attempts she looked at me and then, with a gesture of futility, straightened up.

I stared at him. The pity I felt for him was suddenly almost a physical ache. Maybe *not* responding to us was the only way he could exercise some power. After all, not only couldn't he do anything for himself, he was even helpless against us, couldn't even stop us from treating him if he wanted to.

I also became fully aware, as though for the first time, of how helpless he was against a *sound* that was constantly barraging him—the loud whirring of his bed's motor. I got a radio and turned it on to a station that played soft music. I could only hope that it would override the sound of the motor—and would help soothe him.

A few days later, while giving him his morning care, I noticed that his body tensed and his breathing quickened. This had never happened before; he'd never indicated in any way that he felt anything. I spoke to his doctor about it, told him I was sure it meant my moving and touching him was hurting him.

"No," he said, "he'd have reacted more than

that. He'd have gestured, let out a sound—something."

Angry, frustrated, I watched the doctor walk off. The next day, while I was bathing Mr. Bowen, he stiffened once more. Again I talked to his doctor.

"Doctor, I know what I see. The man hurts. He needs something for pain."

The doctor looked at me, then away, debating with himself. Then he walked over to the nurses' station and wrote out an order for a p.r.n. pain medication.

Before doing Mr. Bowen's morning care the next day, I explained that the needle I was giving him would make it less painful. This time his body remained relaxed; his breathing stayed even.

I hoped that this would be a breakthrough, that perhaps he would trust me enough now to communicate with me in some way. But whatever he felt, he still didn't even acknowledge my presence.

By now a month had passed. In all this time he hadn't had a single visitor. A sister called twice to see how he was, but this was the only trace of interest his family showed in him. Maybe the fact that he seemed so alone, though, helped keep me trying to reach him when, in fact, I had no reason to believe I ever could.

Each morning I continued to announce the day of the week, to talk about the weather. And I would chat as I worked, telling Mr. Bowen things I'd read in the paper or had seen on TV. Whenever I could,

I would sit down and read parts of the newspaper to him, perhaps the major headlines or a humorous story that caught my attention, often some items from the sports pages.

On one such day, about 6 weeks after Mr. Bowen became my patient, I put down the paper, stood up from the chair, and took his hand before leaving. I said—as I had so many times before—"I've got to go check on my other patients now. I'll see you a little later, all right?"

I squeezed his hand. And then—it almost took my breath away—he squeezed back!

Later, when I returned to his room, he did another exciting thing—he turned his head in my direction as soon as he heard my footsteps. During the days that followed, he began to move his arms. He also started nodding his head slightly when I said good morning, and more often than not, he would squeeze my hand in response to a question. His level of alertness increased so that we could generally tell, just by looking at him, if he were asleep or awake.

And he remained responsive even as he began to fail, physically, in the next weeks.

I came in one morning to learn that Mr. Bowen had died. Although it wasn't entirely unexpected, I still felt a small rush of sadness. But it was more for his suffering in the past than for his death. Finally, he was at peace. And I began to feel a kind of peace remembering that squeeze of a hand that told me he knew he was no longer alone.

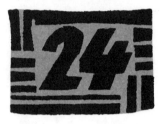

How Could Patti, 20 and Newly Married, Ever Face a Colostomy?

DOLORES ZOPF, RN

Sometimes in dealing with a patient, the nurse has to be alert to a special clock. This is the inner timepiece that signals when to stop immediately... wait awhile... or go ahead now... in her work with a patient. It was this signal we kept watching for with Patti.

Fair-skinned, green-eyed, blond, vivacious, and recently married, Patti was a most attractive 20-year-old. She was also a victim of Crohn's disease.

Typically, this disease of the small intestine mainly attacks young adults. Emotional stress is thought to be a contributing factor. Its insidious process begins at the ileum and causes edema, constriction of the lumen, and crampy abdominal pains. It creates an irritating discharge that empties into the colon and precipitates frequent bouts of diarrhea. The colon becomes inflamed and abscesses form throughout the colon, rectum, and perineal area.

Over the years, Patti had been prescribed palliative diet, rest, and medication. But this had failed to halt the disease, and she'd been hospitalized at least five times. Between hospitalizations, she'd required frequent office consultations

for diarrhea, fever, nausea, vomiting and repeated perineal abscesses.

When we first met, Patti had again been hospitalized for a painful labial abscess. During this period, I got to know her and about her background.

The youngest of five and clearly the family's pet, Patti, possibly because of her illness, was excessively dependent on her mother. Patti's entire family was unhappy when she eloped and married against their wishes because they felt she had "married beneath herself." This show of independence was especially calamitous to her widowed mother, who seemed to need Patti's dependence on her. The relationship between the girl's family and her husband was, on the surface, polite but anyone could see the tension there. And, despite their obvious love for one another, we could also sense a certain malaise between the young couple. They were so young to be faced with such grave problems. Because of Patti's abscesses, sexual intercourse must have been a rare experience for them.

When the abscess finally broke and drained and

Patti was ready to go home, the doctors told her that these debilitating attacks would continue to a point where they would become life-threatening. The only known cure, they said, would be ileostomy. She was discharged for 1 month to consider this grave step.

Our area has a wonderful Ostomy Club, so we asked them to contact Patti. The first volunteers were a young married couple who hoped to talk to Patti and her husband as people in parallel circumstances. Unfortunately, Patti's mother stayed throughout the entire visit, inhibiting the discussion. Patti's second visitor from the Club was a woman in her sixties. Because of the vast difference in their ages, Patti was unable to relate well to her. During this period of decision, Patti again developed an abscess extending into the labia.

Perhaps this was a turning point, because Patti decided to have the operation. She reappeared at our hospital a month later. I should say again "made an appearance" because Patti, in a stunning, bare midriff, two-piece slack suit, emerald green to match her eyes, came on like the most carefree butterfly on the social circuit. Overly exuberant, laughing gaily at anything and everything, presented an unreal picture of a young woman about to undergo a most drastic procedure. Surgery was scheduled for early the next day. But all during the routines of drawing blood, collecting urine samples and taking X-rays, the unnatural party-like atmosphere continued.

Reality was inescapable, however, and early the next morning Patti finally broke. Through sobs she called out, "Oh God, please, God, isn't there some other way? I will never be like anyone else again. What will my husband say when he sees that awful mess on my stomach? Oh God, why me?"

I was assigned to Patti that day. Because of some experiences in my own life, I've probably read and thought more about body image than the average nurse. Any major change in body image is traumatic, I know, but change in the face or torso (which are considered the "essential me"—the core of the person) is much more threatening than change connected with an appendage.

I thought back on this, on all the literature I'd read, and on my own personal experiences. But I couldn't think of a single thing to ease Patti's suffering. She was right to want to be young and

beautiful when she *was* young and beautiful. The operation *was* going to make her "different" from the normal person. And it *was* a cruel decision she had to make. So I just sat quietly beside her bed. Patti continued crying and talking out all her conflicting feelings. Finally, emotionally drained, she rested her head on her pillow indicating that she didn't want to talk any more.

I discussed Patti's outburst with the doctor. After a while he went and talked to her at length. But in the end, Patti had to face it alone; she went to surgery looking as though her world had ended.

Our Director of Nursing called a conference to

Overly exuberant, laughing gaily at anything and everything, Patti presented an unreal picture of a young woman about to undergo a most drastic procedure. Reality was inescapable, however, and early the next morning Patti finally broke.

pool all our information on this case. We discussed the disease, surgery, body image and the emotional tangle of Patti, her husband and her family. Our consensus was to encourage the husband to participate more fully in Patti's care; foster a healthful interdependence between the mother and daughter; and most important, let the patient set her own pace for recovery.

Patti returned from the operating room with an ileostomy located in the right lower quadrant of the abdomen. The first day, we gave her standard postoperative treatment.

The second day, we had her dangle her feet at the side of the bed three times. She needed much encouragement to move and begged us not to make her look at her abdomen.

While standing on the third day, the ileostomy bag became slightly loosened. She cried out in panic, "Please don't make me see it. Oh, God, how awful I smell." Quickly I helped her to bed and just as quickly, I changed the bag.

Finally, on the fourth day while I was changing the dressing, she ventured a quick look at her abdomen. It made her gasp. "Oh, how ugly I am. I hate myself." And she started to cry. But she had made the move... she had looked.

Not wanting to lose this moment, I assured her that the stoma was small, that it would likely get smaller, and that diet and deodorant pills would control odors. I felt sure that in time she would become accustomed to it. "It would take me hours to do what you're doing now," she protested. I explained that she would begin by choosing a quiet time of day when she was unhurried and in a very short time she would be very adept. But that was as much as she could handle for the time. "I'll never care for that thing," she declared and turned away.

Despite this, I was encouraged. She had looked at herself. She had listened. She had considered self-care.

In the meantime, we found opportunity to talk to the husband. He seemed relieved to know that

 She was right to want to be young and beautiful when she was young and beautiful. The operation was going to make her "different" from the normal person.

we had understood the situation between him and Patti's mother. He did want to work more closely in caring for his wife. What he was hoping was that Patti's family would visit during the day so

he and Patti could be alone during the nighttime visiting hours. We decided to present this idea to the family.

Patti's mother proved to be approachable, too. She realized that her own need to be depended upon was causing emotional stress for Patti. She gave up insisting that Patti stay with her until complete recovery, and agreed that upon discharge, Patti would stay with her only 1 week before returning home. The mother would then visit to help with meals and housekeeping until Patti regained her strength.

As several more days passed, Patti continued to be withdrawn and unable to accept the reality of her situation, so we recontacted the Ostomy Club.

Barbara, the young wife who had originally visited Patti, came again. She was an excellent choice. Barbara was 25, attractive and full of life. After her ileostomy, she had several children by normal delivery. Not only was she happy with her life but, most important for Patti to understand, she was happy with herself.

She talked intimately with Patti, displaying her own appliance and also explaining its care and reliving her feelings about it when she was fresh from surgery. Here was someone who knew exactly how Patti was feeling. She agreed to return as often as Patti wanted her.

There was no mistaking the good effects of Barbara's visit, so we decided to reinforce them immediately. We'd noticed that Patti's spirits were very low in the morning, but by afternoon, though still depressed, she seemed stronger, better able to cope. So, we decided to postpone her care until the afternoons when she might be more able to deal with it.

The next morning, instead of giving ostomy care, we just sat and talked, the talk quite naturally turning to the operation. I reintroduced the positive aspects. We compared what her life had been like to what it would be like.

Aside from the basic fact that she could have died from the unchecked Crohn's disease, she could now be in control of her life. She'd be able to go out in public, hold a job, do the housewifely things she loved, without fear of a humiliating and painful bout of cramping diarrhea, nausea, vomiting. She'd no longer require bedrest to restore her from the debilitating effects of these attacks. She'd now be able to sit normally in a chair instead of balancing on one hip because of the painful perineal abscesses. She'd no longer have to wear peri-pads for the foul-smelling drainage from the abscesses. Once healed, she could resume sexual relations with the husband she loved. All these things I said—but were they getting through?

As we talked, I thought I got that signal that said "now." Taking a deep breath, I told her she had to decide whether she was going to involve herself in her own life or waste it mourning what could not be. I reminded her that she was leaving us soon and she really hadn't faced up to herself or her ileostomy. I told her I would be back later to help *her* with her ostomy care.

I admit I was trembling when I left that room. Suppose I had intimidated her by my bluntness? Suppose she decided not to try?

When I returned that afternoon, we decided to change her bag while she was sitting up. As usual, I was explaining what I was doing. While wiping the stoma, I was stressing the need to be gentle, when suddenly her hand, holding a tissue, brushed past mine covering the stoma. "Like this?" she said. Not daring to speak, I nodded my head. Next she applied pressure to the karaya ring, asking if that was the proper way to do it. I said it was, and realized we were both smiling. I felt I had just welcomed her back to life.

Yet, things were not all sunshine and flowers from then on. There were moments when her spirit faltered. The idea of a tub bath made her panicky. She shuddered to think that the bag might come off and spill the contents into the water. I told her it wasn't likely but if it did happen, we'd just change the water, put on another bag and continue with the shampoo and bath. The bag didn't come off, but she still resisted the idea of the tubs despite the doctor's explaining how it was helping to heal the perineal abscesses.

On the third day of doing her own care, Patti stated that she minded the ileostomy care less than looking at the suture line. This seemed encouraging.

Little by little, Patti moved toward discharge and total independence. And as we watched, we were glad we had waited and let her face up to her new life in her own time.

Dr. Evans, Obsessed with Food, Was Starving Himself

IRENE M. MISIK, RN, BSN

One of the first lessons a psychiatric nurse learns is: *Don't expect too much from your patients.* Still, no matter how often we remind ourselves of this lesson, we usually have to relearn it with every difficult patient we care for.

Dr. Richard Evans had anorexia nervosa, and he didn't even *want* to get well. What's more, with his medical background—he was a dentist—he knew exactly how to *keep* from getting well.

When 48-year-old Dr. Evans admitted himself to our short-term psychiatric unit, he weighed only 96 pounds (43.2 kg)—and he was 6 feet 2 inches (185 cm) tall. This was his first admission to a psychiatric unit. According to his records, his adult weight had been 140 pounds (63 kg) until age 45. Then he'd become involved in a costly divorce suit, and his weight had plummeted to under 100 pounds (45 kg).

Besides anorexia, Dr. Evans also had prerenal azotemia (an excess of nitrogenous bodies in the blood), diffuse kidney damage, and edema. The doctors suspected diuretic abuse. So besides a weight-gaining regimen and psychotherapy, the doctors planned to restrict his fluid intake, put him on a salt-free diet, and use diuretics in controlled amounts.

Since most anorectics are female adolescents, Dr. Evans was an unusual case. But his way of dealing with his illness—denial—wasn't unusual at all.

During my nursing assessment, Dr. Evans first told me he had a "dread fear" of weight gain and had to force himself to eat. Then, almost in the same breath, he denied it. He said that his weight loss wasn't a problem, that he was simply "too busy and too nervous to eat."

Although Dr. Evans was pitifully emaciated, feeling sympathetic toward him was difficult. During our conversation, he was standoffish, and his eyes were, frankly, unfriendly.

Since the hospital where I work is one of the biggest centers in the country for treating anorexia nervosa, we've all cared for dozens of anorectic patients. As charge nurse on the evening shift, I've cared for at least 50 myself. Still, every time we admit another, we prepare ourselves for the worst, because in our experience, no patients are as manipulative and demanding as these. We had hoped, though, that Dr. Evans might be less difficult than most. After all, with his medical background, wouldn't he be more receptive to our care plan?

Not necessarily. But we didn't find out just how *unreceptive* he was for a few days.

Since we weren't sure how closely he'd have to be supervised, we first let Dr. Evans eat in the patients' dining room. We asked the nursing assistant who monitored the dining room to discreetly observe Dr. Evans' eating behavior. She reported nothing out of the ordinary until the third day, when she realized Dr. Evans had been craftily chewing his food and spitting it out.

He'd remove the lid from his plate, select a piece of food, chew it thoroughly, and then spit it out and carefully replace the lid on the plate. He repeated this procedure until he'd chewed everything on his plate. Yet, at the end of a meal, he probably hadn't swallowed more than a few bites.

I observed this for myself. "Is something wrong with your food?" I asked, sitting next to him. "Too much fat," Dr. Evans said. I lifted the lid on his plate, trying to control my nausea. "That looks like more than fat to me," I said. But he insisted he was eating everything but the fat.

The other patients began complaining. How could they eat with Dr. Evans in the same room? We asked the nursing assistant to sit with him during meals, but he continued to spit out his food.

After a week, we started serving Dr. Evans his meals in his room—unsupervised. We knew he resented being treated like a child, and we thought that if we left him alone he'd begin eating more normally. We also asked him to begin recording his food and fluid intake, hoping that the responsibility of recording his intake would make him more compliant to his regimen.

The dietitian discussed his food preferences with him and tried to include his favorite foods in his daily menu. But even though Dr. Evans ordered huge amounts of food, he continued to chew his food and then spit it out, so his plates were always just as full *after* he'd eaten as before. And he always recorded everything he ordered as intake, even though it was never "in" very long. Needless to say, determining Dr. Evans' caloric intake was impossible.

Like many anorectics, Dr. Evans was preoccupied with food even though he rarely ate. Shortly after we began serving him his meals in his room, the other patients complained that dishes of food were missing from their trays. At first, we thought the dietary department had made a mistake, but then we found several containers of uneaten food in the unit's refrigerator. Each container was marked "Dr. Richard Evans." Dr. Evans denied stealing the food, claiming that someone must be trying to get him in trouble.

Denial, Dr. Evans' response to any challenging statement from us, also served as a defense mechanism to help him deal with anxiety. So we didn't want to destroy this coping mechanism.

On the other hand, we didn't want him to think he'd pulled the wool over our eyes, either. So every time he denied something, we'd present him with the evidence and tell him that we knew he was denying. But he'd always fix his unfriendly eyes on us and then walk away in a huff. We might as well have been talking to a wall.

One day, Dr. Evans carried denial to the outer limits. We'd told him he wasn't allowed in the kitchen, but we'd often catch him with his head in the refrigerator. This time, though, we caught him red-handed with a glass of juice.

"You know you're not allowed any more fluids today," I scolded. "Who's drinking?" Dr. Evans said, between gulps of juice.

Dr. Evans had been our patient for 2 weeks, and he was *losing* weight instead of gaining it. He was down to 85 pounds (38.3 kg), and his behavior was getting more bizarre every day.

He was fanatical about exercising, and we *literally* had to pull him off the exercise bicycle, or he'd ride for hours. An orderly found him drinking water during his shower. A nurse found him eating toothpaste. When we checked the label on the toothpaste, we learned it had a high sodium content. Dr. Evans had told us repeatedly that he was afraid of getting edema, yet he obviously took sodium to promote it.

The last straw came 3 weeks after Dr. Evans' admission. At this point, I think *we* were losing weight from all the exercise we got following him around. We searched his room because we suspected he was hiding forbidden medications.

Sure enough, we found three full dispensing bottles of diuretics, and a cache of sodium saccharin packets. But he'd also hoarded all sorts of hospital supplies: towels, bed linens, soap, tooth-paste. We also found cartons of juice and con-tainers of uneaten, rotting food.

None of us could remember ever being so angry with a patient. Dr. Evans, now down to 79 pounds (35.6 kg), was ordered to a medical unit for hy-peralimentation.

Frankly, we were relieved to see him go, and Dr. Evans, surprisingly, seemed quite content when

 Like many anorectics, Dr. Evans was preoccupied with food even though he rarely ate. Shortly after we began serving him his meals in his room, the other patients complained that dishes of food were missing from their trays. "You know you're not allowed any more fluids today," I scolded. "Who's drinking?" Dr. Evans said, between gulps of juice.

we visited him. "Something's wrong with my body, you see. *That's* why I can't eat," he told us right-eously. He seemed to enjoy the "sick" role, be-cause he could blame his problems on something physical, therefore, out of his hands.

After 3 weeks of hyperalimentation, Dr. Evans had gained 23 pounds (10.4 kg). We were en-couraged and discouraged at the same time. After all, what kind of "progress" is *losing* 17 pounds (7.7 kg) and then gaining back 23 (10.4 kg)?

To steel ourselves for Dr. Evans' return, we held a staff conference to draw up a contract. We'd

used contracts before with anorectics who weren't complying, but since contracts are so restrictive, we use them only as a last resort. But with Dr. Evans, we had no choice. And if the contract didn't work, we didn't know what we'd do.

When we presented the contract to Dr. Evans, he accused us of running the unit like a Boy Scout camp. But we finally convinced him to sign the document.

We assigned a nursing assistant to stay with Dr. Evans whenever he was out of his room—not just at mealtimes. Then we assigned *two* assistants to supervise him during meals. This way, if he tried to manipulate one assistant, she'd have a witness to back her up. We hated to monitor Dr. Evans so closely, and we knew he'd hate it, too. We hoped he'd hate it enough to start cooperating.

We decided on another way to reward Dr. Evans for acceptable behavior. Unlike most of our pa-tients, he was comfortable in a leadership role. To reward him, we'd let him lead our informal patient discussion groups. If he didn't comply with his contract, he'd lose his leadership privileges.

When we told Dr. Evans about being supervised during meals, he was indignant. But when we told him he could earn the privilege of being a group leader, he seemed interested. Not pleased. That would've been asking too much of Dr. Evans. His exact response was, "I don't know why you waited so long to ask me."

The first time Dr. Evans led a discussion, he even managed to persuade some of our more with-drawn patients to talk about themselves. But when he started giving lectures on exercise and nutrition, we became a little concerned. Amazingly, how-ever, he gave *good* advice. He certainly didn't practice what he preached, but he obviously knew his stuff.

The discussion groups also gave Dr. Evans an opportunity to vent some of his feelings. We had three other anorectics on our unit, and Dr. Evans was convinced that we were treating them better than him. We don't usually encourage anorectics to talk with one another, because they often swap "diet" hints. But we wanted Dr. Evans to deal with his anger maturely, so we suggested that he con-front the other patients with his complaints.

"You're not obeying the rules like I am," he told them. One girl responded by telling him to take a good look at himself. "You're still skinny as a stick, but I'm gaining weight," she said. Dr. Evans looked offended, but hearing a criticism from another anorectic seemed therapeutic. Later on, he actually confessed, "I guess my diet isn't as good as it should be."

Although Dr. Evans still looked for loopholes in his contract and still tried to manipulate us, he wasn't as devious as before. Passing the 100-pound (45-kg) mark must've been a milestone for him. Now, he seemed to accept the inevitability of gaining weight, and most days he achieved his 4-pound (0.2-kg) weight gain. Eventually, he stopped ordering enormous meals and stopped stealing and hoarding food. But most important, he stopped spitting out his food. He wasn't exactly a glutton, but at least he was swallowing.

We told him how well he looked and how pleased we were with his progress. We also told him we thought he was doing a good job leading the discussion groups. If he appreciated our compliments, we'll never know. He remained aloof and unapproachable all during his illness.

After 3 months on our unit, Dr. Evans weighed 124 pounds (55.8 kg), and we all agreed that he was as ready for discharge as he'd ever be. When we told him he'd be discharged soon, we were encouraged by his response: He immediately began discussing a reasonable career change. He thought he'd like to turn to health care administration.

We helped him schedule job interviews and gave him all the moral support we could. Our dietitian helped him plan menus, and we arranged for him to weigh in with us once a week. His psychiatrist scheduled him on an outpatient basis.

Although I never saw Dr. Evans again, the nurses on the day shift saw him every time he came to the unit to be weighed. They said he was just as unapproachable as ever, but that he seemed to have his anorexia under control. In fact, he'd even gained another 10 pounds (4.5 kg).

I thought over what the nurses said, and I think I recognize one big mistake we made with Dr. Evans. Our mistake *wasn't* in the kind of care we gave him. After all, he'd started eating again and had gained 28 pounds (12.6 kg)—exactly what he'd come into the hospital to achieve. Our mistake was in expecting him to react to our care and concern the way patients normally do. But what's normal for one person isn't always normal for another.

At his best, Dr. Evans was probably always a difficult, unbending person—and we couldn't change that. But we *did* help him change from what he was at his worst—devious, manipulative, and self-destructive.

Cal Wanted to Take Charge

CAROL TEA, RN

As a new nurse on a rehabilitation unit, I'd thought a lot about *accepting* responsibility. But I'd never thought about *abdicating* it—until I met Cal, a 29-year-old quadriplegic.

Cal had become a quadriplegic 2 years before, after a motorcycle accident. Since then, he'd been in and out of hospitals and had had many complications, including bowel and bladder incontinence, urinary tract infections, and draining sacral and trochanteric decubiti.

When I learned Cal would be my first primary care patient, I was both eager and a little awed. I knew his physical care alone would be a big job— the feeding, bathing, bowel training program, and so on. But I had other goals, too: to help him accept his altered body image and to help him prepare for the future. Until he was ready to resume control, *I'd* be responsible for his welfare.

"Don't worry," I lectured myself, "It's a big responsibility, but you're perfectly capable."

Only when the aide wheeled Cal into his room, though, did I really appreciate the magnitude of my responsibility. Eighty-four vital pounds (37.8 kg) barely covered Cal's 6-foot (180-cm) frame.

His arms and legs were severely contracted, with only trace bicep activity in his right arm.

But his eyes were alive, and they surveyed the ward with eager curiosity. During my nursing assessment, Cal exuded optimism.

"When can I get started? How can I help? What equipment do I need?" His enthusiasm was infectious, and obviously he had high hopes. *I* had high hopes, too, and I couldn't wait to begin working with him.

Cal's contractures were so bad that he couldn't bend at the hips to sit up. So my first effort was to increase his strength and reduce the contractures in his legs and hips by doing range-of-motion exercises. The first day I raised the head of his bed 5° and kept it at this angle for 5 minutes. Every few days I raised the bed 5° more and increased the time by 5 minutes. Slowly but surely Cal's tolerance and strength increased, and we worked our way toward our goal—sitting upright. Then, boom—Cal got a urinary tract infection and was so ill he was flat on his back again.

The same thing happened with the range-of-motion exercises for his arms. Since Cal *could* tense the muscles in his right arm and shoulder, I worked especially hard to strengthen those muscles. But just when we began to see some progress, Cal got another infection, and we were back at square one.

Cal's enthusiasm waned with every setback. In the beginning, he'd been so eager and hopeful about rehabilitation—but perhaps he'd expected too much too soon. The almost constant urinary tract infections were getting him down—physically *and* emotionally—and his behavior changed dramatically. Before his injury he'd been a sergeant in the army, and now he took command, ordering me and the other nurses around as if we were in boot camp.

If we failed to answer his call light within 5 seconds, he screamed at the top of his lungs. If he didn't get two full packs of cigarettes a day, he dressed us down for unfair treatment. And if we didn't turn him every 2 hours *on the dot,* he accused us of purposely neglecting him.

Worse yet, many of Cal's orders were based on partial understanding or misinformation. For instance, he believed that the way to prevent a urinary tract infection was to drink as much as possible. So he begged fluids from staff, housekeeping, and well-meaning friends, until his intake reached 10 liters a day.

What's more, like most spinal cord injured patients, Cal had a lot of sediment in his urine, and when the sediment built up inside the catheter, the urine couldn't drain properly. And obviously, drinking 10 liters of fluids daily only made the problem worse. Cal grew even thinner and weaker from lack of appetite, his bladder became distended, urine leaked around his Foley catheter, and his decubiti became contaminated. Needless to say, bladder management was nearly impossible, and my whole rehabilitation program came to a screeching halt.

Finally, the doctors removed Cal's Foley and tried an external condom catheter, hoping that it would cut down on the number of urinary tract infections. Unfortunately, when Cal's bladder got too full, the force of the urine flow popped the catheter off, creating new problems. Still, the advantages outweighed the problems, so we put up with occasional "accidents," all the while trying to persuade Cal to stop overloading his bladder.

But no one could convince him that he needed *less* fluids, not *more*. I drew diagrams of the urinary system and showed him his intake and output records. Nothing helped. So *we* started issuing commands, strictly monitoring his fluid intake and posting signs around his room asking visitors not to give him anything to drink. But when Cal's urinary tract infections didn't disappear immediately, he blamed *us*—because we hadn't followed *his* orders.

While Cal vacillated between angry outbursts and days of silent withdrawal, my neat care plan became a shambles. Still I didn't give up. Since Cal complained constantly about hospital food, to coax him to eat I brought milkshakes from fast-food restaurants and added a high-protein mixture. He just turned up his nose. I spent even more time explaining every procedure to him, but he told me he already knew everything and then informed me that my way of doing things was wrong.

At the end of one long day, the charge nurse asked me to "do something with Cal." For some reason, that day he was *refusing* liquids and also refusing medications. Wearily, I went to talk with him.

Grim-lipped, Cal told me he intended to refuse all medications, fluids, and treatments until he got what he wanted—more diazepam (Valium). Patiently, I restated all the reasons why he should take his medications and the consequences of his persistent noncompliance.

Finally he thundered, "I *have* to refuse everything! My mouth is my only control."

In the silence that followed, I began to understand that my plan for taking care of Cal had excluded his need to take care of *himself*. I'd been planning everything *for* him, making him a passive recipient. And at this stage—rehabilitation—Cal didn't need to be on the receiving end only; he needed to take charge.

"Okay, Cal, you're right," I said. "A lot of your control *does* come from your mouth. But you've also got a brain in your head, and you know that what you're doing isn't in your best interests. Still, it's your choice. You can have one problem, the need for Valium, or *two* problems: the need for Valium and an uncontrolled urinary tract infection. It's up to you."

The next morning, I learned that Cal had taken

all his medications without complaining. I also learned that, after 6 months on our unit, Cal had been transferred to an acute care hospital for excision of a kidney abscess—the source of his urinary tract infections.

My problems with Cal weren't gone forever—I knew he'd be readmitted. But one of the beauties of rehabilitation nursing is that it's an ongoing process, giving a nurse time to develop a trusting relationship with her patients. So I used the interval as a respite, to reorganize a better approach to Cal's care. Next time around he'd have a *say* in his care plan.

When Cal returned, I was ready. I showed him the Kardex and explained how we nurses used it as a communication tool.

"What are you going to write about me?" he asked.

"This is *your* plan for rehabilitation, Cal," I said. "So let's start with what's important to you."

The life I'd seen in his eyes that first day sparked again. "I want to take a car trip across the United States," he said.

They say the longest journey begins with a single step, and Cal and I sat through the afternoon planning. So far, all our goals had been short-term—like increasing his strength so he could sit up. But now we had a *long-range* goal to work for, and that seemed to make all the difference—to both of us. I told Cal we had a lot of work to do before his trip. We had to build up his tolerance for sitting, increase his overall strength, and start a bladder management program. I even reminded him that he'd be eating in fast-food chains all across the country, so he'd better stop turning up his nose at hospital food.

Cal and I began our exercise program again. With the urinary tract infections under control, we made slow but steady progress with graduated sitting and range-of-motion exercises. To record his progress, I posted weight charts at his bedside and filled in the weight as he gained it. Then we drew up a contract—a two-column chart that indicated both the staff's and Cal's responsibilities.

At the top of the contract was the activity that had been one of our first sources of conflict—regular turning. On the staff side of the contract I wrote: "Turn every 2 hours," and then I added a proviso for 15 minutes' leeway. And on Cal's side I wrote, "Assist with every turn."

Now that Cal was taking part in his own care, we needed some devices to help him be more mobile and more independent. A "friction mitt," worn like a glove, allowed him to push the wheel of his wheelchair, and a "bath mitt," slipped on his hand, helped him wash himself. To prevent his legs from contracting when he was lying down, I invented a foam rubber device, $30 \times 30 \times 3$ inches $(75 \times 75 \times 7.5$ cm$)$. I wrapped the foam around Cal's legs and tied it in place with stockinette to keep his legs extended.

But the device that gave Cal the most independence was a tenodesis splint. The splint fit around his right wrist and the second and third fingers of his right hand, with wires connecting the wrist and finger pieces. When Cal hyperextended his wrist, his thumb and fingers pinched together, allowing him to pick things up. With the splint on, he could feed himself, and he could even, I hoped, catheterize himself.

When I told Cal I wanted him to learn self-catheterization, he eagerly accepted the challenge.

One of the beauties of rehabilitation nursing is that it's an ongoing process, giving a nurse time to develop a trusting relationship with her patients.

At one point, Cal's scrupulous attention to detail had been a problem; now it was an important part of his coping skills. I wrote out the steps for self-catheterization and posted them at Cal's bedside, and Cal painstakingly memorized each step.

Cal's sharp eyes helped him identify problems and confront them before they became overwhelming. He had trouble reaching the catheterization equipment on his bedside table, so he decided to store the supplies in a lazy Susan. Then he could rotate the lazy Susan until the piece of equipment he needed was within reach. He also discovered that a silverware organizer was a good container for storing and soaking catheters.

Learning self-catheterization was exhausting for Cal, but he never gave up, even though the procedure took him 1½ hours at first. I'd position the tenodesis splint for him, and then he'd slip it onto his right hand. He'd take a washcloth from the lazy Susan, wipe his hands and penis, and prop up his penis with the washcloth. Then he'd take the catheter out of the silverware organizer and put the tip into a jar of lubricating jelly.

To make this last step easier, I stretched a rubber glove over the top of the jar, secured the glove with a rubber band, and then cut a hole in the middle of the glove. That way, when Cal withdrew the catheter from the jar, excess jelly stayed in the jar.

Last, Cal would insert the catheter into his bladder and drain the urine into a urine-collection box. I attached a handle to the box so he could slip his arm through the handle to pick up the box.

After several weeks of practicing, Cal had the entire procedure down to 6 minutes.

As Cal made strides toward independence, I realized I'd been stifling him like an over-protec-tive mother. So I created a little invention of my own, a form of behavior modification. I slipped a rubber band around my wrist and every time I caught myself playing mother hen, I'd snap the rubber band as a reminder.

The months passed, and Cal and I changed and grew. Although no miracles happened, and we both had setbacks, eventually Cal was wheeling himself around the unit and taking care of many of his own needs.

After 14 months, Cal was discharged to a transitional living center while his house was adapted for wheelchair accessibility. He finished a driver's education course and *did* make that long-awaited car trip, accompanied by a friend. Now he's studying computer technology.

In retrospect, I can see that my original care plan was directed too much toward me. I'd assumed I could take full responsibility for Cal's welfare, and then, when *I* thought he was ready, I'd let him take care of himself. And Cal had assumed that he was ready to take care of himself from the start.

Sometimes, taking responsibility for a patient's welfare is the easiest part of rehabilitative nursing. The hardest part is giving that responsibility *back*.

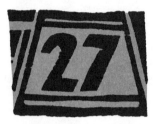

To Punish Herself, Laura Mutilated Her Body

KAREN R. PALERMO, RN, BSN

As psychiatric nurses, we've been taught to *expect* some patients to be difficult. But sometimes, "difficult" is the wrong word—"impossible" is more like it. Take Laura, for instance. We had to watch her constantly to keep her from destroying herself.

Twenty-three-year-old Laura was admitted to our surgical unit after deliberately swallowing a spoon. Hoping the spoon would eventually be eliminated naturally, the surgeon decided not to operate. Two days later, Laura was transferred to the mental health unit where I work.

When I learned I'd be Laura's primary care nurse, I reviewed her chart. As a child, she'd been tied to a chair and beaten by her father. When she was 16, she'd started a series of self-mutilations that had kept her in and out of mental institutions ever since.

The doctors diagnosed her illness as "borderline personality organization"—a type of schizophrenia that manifests itself in depression, rage, panic, guilt, passivity, and helplessness.

In the midst of my reading, I heard a quiet voice say, "Nurse, could I please have some medicine? I've got awful pain."

I glanced up and saw a slender, blond young woman—Laura. I introduced myself and told her she wasn't due for pain medication for 30 minutes. Her face fell in disappointment, but then she shrugged her shoulders and walked away. Her thin, short-sleeved dress didn't hide the terrible scars on her arms and legs. She looked as if she'd been caught in a fire.

And she *had*. But every fire Laura'd been caught in had been set by Laura. For 7 years, she'd been punishing herself by burning her body and by forcing spoons down her throat. Looking at Laura's body was like reading her autobiography—every burn, every scar, signifying a battle with herself—a battle lost.

Laura also had a seizure disorder, but daily doses of phenobarbital and phenytoin sodium (Dilantin) were controlling the seizures.

I was about to give Laura her medication when I heard a crash and a continuous dull thumping. I found Laura thrashing on the hall floor—obviously having a grand mal seizure. Quickly, I put a tongue blade in her mouth, turned her head and body to one side, and called for help.

When the doctor arrived, Laura's seizure was over. He ordered a blood test, and the test showed almost nonexistent levels of anticonvulsant medication. No wonder Laura'd had a seizure.

"Laura, have you just been *pretending* to swallow your medicine?" I asked. "The voices told me not to take it," she replied.

The doctor ordered a *stat* dose of phenobarbital and placed Laura on complete bed rest. Over the next few days, I made sure she was getting her medicine, checking inside her mouth to make sure she'd swallowed the pills. But even with the medication, she had seizures every 4 or 5 hours, around the clock.

"I think I'm going to have a seizure. Get a tongue blade quick," Laura'd yell, sending us scrambling. Then, sometimes she'd have a seizure, and sometimes she wouldn't.

Then we noticed something odd about her seizures. For one thing, they continued even after her medication reached therapeutic levels. And while she was convulsing, she pulled in her tongue and turned her body to one side. She never frothed at the mouth, and her skin color and vital signs remained normal.

So we called in a neurologist. After one of Laura's seizures, the doctor held her eyes open and moved a mirror back and forth in front of her face. Her eyes followed the mirror. "She's faking," he said.

Knowing Laura was faking was little comfort for us. We couldn't simply ignore her seizure threats—suppose some time she really *did* have a seizure? So we held a staff meeting to discuss how to ensure Laura's safety without reinforcing her attention-getting behavior.

One of the nurses suggested having Laura wear a football helmet. Since we couldn't watch her constantly, the helmet would protect her head if she had a real seizure and, we hoped, would discourage her from faking. Ironically, Laura was vain about her appearance, and we suspected she'd hate the helmet.

Just as we'd suspected, Laura hated the bulky, bright orange helmet. She whined constantly—she couldn't eat, couldn't see, and the other patients were staring at her because she looked foolish. "When your seizures stop, we'll take it off," we told her. And, in a few days, her seizures stopped.

But we knew a football helmet wouldn't cure all Laura's problems. Now that she wasn't getting extra attention, she became even more demanding. She camped at the nurses' station, tugging at our uniforms and pleading for attention. Every sentence started with "I want." We set firm limits— if she wanted to talk, we'd be glad to talk—in 10 minutes. Obviously hurt and angry, Laura began dividing us into "good" and "bad" nurses. Manipulation was Laura's strong point, and she actually succeeded in creating bad feelings among the staff.

"Last night I felt like hurting myself," she'd tell me. "But Mary said she was too busy to help me." At first, I was angry. How could Mary ignore Laura when she was crying for help? But when I

Obviously hurt and angry, Laura began dividing us into "good" and "bad" nurses. Manipulation was Laura's strong point, and she actually succeeded in creating bad feelings among the staff.

confronted Mary, she told me she *hadn't* ignored Laura, and that Laura hadn't said a word about hurting herself.

Other nurses complained of this kind of manipulation, too. So before we ended up at each other's throats, we decided that when Laura told one nurse that another nurse had mistreated her, we'd immediately summon the other nurse. Then the three of us could talk out the problem.

Laura burst into tears when I brought Mary to hear Laura's accusation firsthand. "You ignored me, and I almost swallowed a spoon," Laura said between sobs. "You never said anything about swallowing a spoon," Mary said. "Well, maybe I didn't *say* I wanted to hurt myself, but I *did* want to," Laura whined. "We can't read your mind, Laura," Mary told her.

After several three-way conversations, Laura stopped trying to manipulate us. She simply wasn't getting anywhere, and she knew it. She did, however, continue to have favorite nurses, and she'd play on our sympathy, telling us, in graphic detail, how her father sexually molested her.

We were short-staffed one weekend, about 2 weeks after Laura's admission, and we had several other difficult patients. Laura was especially demanding that weekend, and we were getting short-tempered.

"Why don't you go play cards with the other patients?" I suggested. Laura glared at me and stalked off toward her room. *She'll probably hide under the covers and sulk*, I thought.

A few minutes later, we smelled smoke—the wastebasket in the hall bathroom was on fire. Quickly, we extinguished the flames, then we heard a shriek from Laura's room.

Laura was lying in bed with her nightgown ablaze, and she was screaming in terror. We stripped off the gown and threw it in the sink. Luckily, her burns were only superficial.

Talk about a close call. Maybe Laura'd only wanted to burn herself, but she could've taken everyone in the building with her. Immediately after the doctor treated her burns, we placed Laura in seclusion—for her protection and everyone else's. And because we were afraid she might try to strangle herself with her hospital gown, we restrained her arms. We told her she'd be in seclusion for 12 hours, and even though we'd check on her frequently, she shouldn't expect any special treatment. "We want you to think hard about what you did," we said.

"I couldn't help it," Laura screamed as we fastened the restraints. "The voices made me do it."

We told her *she* was responsible for her actions, and that being in seclusion was her own doing, no one else's.

Laura screamed and screamed for the next few hours. But by the time her seclusion was over, she was screamed out. When we removed the restraints, she just glared at us in contempt.

Once Laura was out of seclusion, we channeled her energies into constructive projects. She liked to cook, so we put her to work in the unit's kitchen,

baking goodies for the patients and staff. Of course, we supervised her whenever she used the stove, and we removed all potentially dangerous kitchen utensils.

Laura baked with a fury, and she was a *good* cook. We praised her lavishly, and every compliment sent her rushing to the kitchen to bake more. Her popularity with the other patients soared. Because she seemed most interested in domestic chores, we asked her if she'd like to help the other patients do their laundry at the neighborhood Laundromat. She enthusiastically agreed. Doing laundry also gave Laura a chance to socialize with the other patients, outside of the hospital. Of course, a staff member always went along.

After 3 weeks in the unit, Laura seemed greatly improved. She still needed constant surveillance, but she hadn't tried to burn herself again, and her threats of "I'm going to hurt myself," had stopped. We were encouraged.

Laura's biggest step forward came when she was elected chairperson of the patient government meeting. Laura was thrilled, but we were wary. Could she handle the responsibility? Or would she try to manipulate the other patients the way she'd tried to manipulate us? Still, we encouraged her, hoping the experience might teach her to be more assertive and less clinging.

Laura led the first meeting skillfully—using perfect parliamentary procedure. The other patients praised her, and we could almost see her self-esteem grow. But then, at the end of the meeting, Laura told Bill, a patient who was about her age, that she liked him and wanted to get to know him better. "Get lost," he said. "I don't like *you* one bit." Poor Laura rushed out of the room in tears, crawled into her bed, and refused to leave it.

When I heard what had happened, I immediately went to talk to her. "No one likes me," she said. "I'm not going to any more meetings."

"But the other patients *do* like you, Laura—that's why they elected you chairperson," I said. Then I explained to her that Bill had his own problems—that a lot of people didn't like *him*, and he'd taken out his anger on her.

We held another staff meeting to decide how to get Laura out of bed and back into the patient community. We could force her to attend the meetings, but we couldn't force her to be chairperson.

We decided to ask the patients to urge her to chair the meetings again.

Laura greeted the other patients by turning her back when they entered her room. She adamantly refused to speak to them. Finally, they left.

Later, when Laura learned they'd elected another chairperson, she was disgusted by how easily they'd replaced her. And she was disgusted with me. "Why didn't you *make* me go to the meeting?" she demanded. I reminded her that *she* was the one who'd chosen not to go.

Then Laura and I discussed her experience with Bill. "Why didn't you stay and confront him?" I asked. After all, she'd been able to confront the "bad" nurses, even though her accusations had been invalid. I told her that this time, she'd had a *valid* reason for a confrontation, and if she'd stayed, I was sure the other patients would've supported her. Laura and I had these talks over several days, and eventually, she got out of bed and joined the meetings again.

We felt more optimistic about Laura's emotional health after she rejoined the patient community, but we didn't feel so optimistic about her physical health. She seemed to be in more pain than usual, and this time, we didn't think she was faking.

When I asked Laura if she felt ill, she tearfully admitted that she'd swallowed three pencils after Bill had insulted her. "I was angry, so I hurt myself," she said. She'd been too ashamed to tell me about it and had been in constant pain for a week.

Although swallowing three pencils was recidivist behavior, Laura's reaction to what she'd done showed progress. This time, she hadn't blamed the "voices," she'd blamed herself. And she wasn't crying for attention or sympathy like before.

Laura had an endoscopy under local anesthesia to remove the pencils, and she cooperated throughout the procedure. Then, because the spoon hadn't passed through her intestine, she was scheduled for a laparotomy. She tolerated this operation well, too.

A few days after her surgery, we started making discharge plans. After 5 weeks in our unit, Laura was transferred to a long-term care facility. We heard that 3 months later she was transferred to a halfway house.

Of course, Laura was far from cured by her stay in our unit, but I *do* feel she took some very positive steps. The most positive step of all came after she swallowed the pencils—when, for the first time, she accepted the responsibility for her actions. For Laura, who'd fought nothing but losing battles with herself, this was not a small victory.

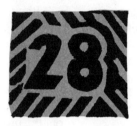

We Had to Help Katie Adjust Her Expectations

LAUREN ELLS, RN

If ever the "herd instinct" is powerful, it's during adolescence. Teenagers hate to be different from their peers. But 13-year-old Katie Richards *was* different because she had a rare, disfiguring disease, arteriovenous malformation of the leg. Guiding her through a long, complicated treatment meant helping her accept one setback after another. It wasn't easy. She was hospitalized for 8 months, and we had to tailor her expectations almost weekly.

Just how tough that would be was clear from the day I stopped by to introduce myself. Although Katie was alone in her semiprivate room, she still kept the bed curtains drawn. Curious, I pulled them back to find her reading a magazine with her head propped up with pillows.

A pretty girl with short brown hair and large, almond-shaped eyes, she was not easy to talk to. In fact, she hardly spoke at all. A sports trophy by her bedside caught my attention, and I thought it might provide the opening I needed. Most kids just love to talk about their accomplishments. But not Katie. The moment I picked up the trophy (which was an award for gymnastics), her eyes started blinking, and I could tell she was fighting

back tears. "Please put that back," she finally said. "It's from last year and I don't know why my parents packed it with my other stuff, anyway."

I knew why and so did she. After a few more minutes of conversation, it became apparent that she wanted to win more trophies—and I soon realized that she expected to start winning them this coming school year. "I came here with two good legs," she said. "And before gym practice starts, I'm going home with two good legs—and nothing and nobody is going to change that."

But I knew changes would have to be made, especially in her attitude. Her expectations were unrealistic because of the vascular disease of her entire left leg. Her condition was serious. She might eventually lose that leg.

Four months before, she'd fractured her left femur in a routine dismount from the parallel bars in her school gym. But her real problem was that the bone had been weakened by arteriovenous malformation (AVM), a disease few of us had ever heard of before. Her AVM had been diagnosed in early childhood. Still, she functioned like most kids her age. But by her 13th birthday, the arteries in her leg had become dangerously distended. Even more alarming, her leg was colored shades of purple and blue. To stop the AVM's invasive growth, her doctors wanted to perform a series of embolizations to diminish the AVM's blood supply.

By now, Katie had become very self-conscious about her appearance, and she always kept her leg hidden under her bed covers. She also instructed her nurses to keep her bed drapes closed at all times.

At her worst, she was withdrawn, but every now and then she would let her true feelings out. "What's going to happen to me, Lauren?" she'd say, almost in tears.

I couldn't tell her because I didn't know myself. But I could help her revise some of her enormous expectations. If hers had been a more predictable illness, a rational discussion about what might happen to her would be easier. But her illness was far from predictable.

To lessen her anxiety, we made out a daily schedule of activities, including times for wake-up, bathing, meals, homework, play, TV, sleep, and physical therapy. The schedule was posted on her wall for quick reference, and we gave copies to the staff school teacher and play therapist so they could cooperate with her when possible. The only time she would leave her room was for her daily physical therapy, which, as an athlete, she loved.

By giving her some control over her life, the schedule worked marvels for motivating her. But it sure caused us a few problems. She used the schedule to control *us*. Let me give you a couple of examples.

To raise her caloric intake, Katie was scheduled to have a milk shake every evening. One night when I brought the shake 2 minutes late, she refused to drink it. *"My* schedule says 9 o'clock sharp," she declared. In other words, she was telling me *It's my way or no way at all*. And once she even refused to take her bath when the nurse wanted to start it a few minutes early.

Some of us put up with her "appointments" good-naturedly, while others were driven to distraction by them. But we all understood this was Katie's way of coping with her doubts and fears while in the hospital.

One week after her admission, the first embolization was performed and she was given pain medications for 2 days afterward. When the pain lessened, she withdrew into herself again. "Team tryouts are next month," she told me almost in a whisper, "and I've got to be there."

Katie went to no tryouts. Instead, she wound up on intravenous (I.V.) antibiotics when she developed septicemia and her second embolization had to be postponed. She reacted to this sudden reversal by blaming her doctors. "Now I've got to spend 3 extra weeks in the hospital doing nothing because of their mistakes," she said.

Once again, her expectations had gotten the best of her, and I made a point of sitting down for a few minutes and explaining that septicemia was a fairly common complication of embolizations. She started to accept the idea that she would miss the tryouts for her school's gymnastics team, but she still didn't relish the idea of staying in the hospital longer than she had planned. "Keep your plans flexible, Katie," I said. "There's no way to know for sure how this will turn out." That was the best advice I gave her.

I decided the surest way to preserve her confidence was to be as honest as I could without being judgmental. She was a teenager, after all, and an athlete. I didn't want her to lose hope—I just wanted her to be open to whatever might happen.

My approach seemed to work. One night, she confided that sometimes she felt as if her leg prevented her from being normal, and being normal was the most important thing to her. That was critical for her to admit because she was telling me how vulnerable she felt. Usually she tried hard to appear strong and unafraid in front of others.

Just how determined she could be was obvious from her progress in physical therapy, where she steadily advanced from the tilt table to the parallel bars. We had never seen such strength of will from an adolescent before. Her emotional outlook began to improve, too. We concentrated on giving her positive feedback, and one day we all were surprised to find her bed curtains open. For the first time in 3 months, Katie actually took an interest in her roommate. She also stopped playing games with us about her inflexible schedule. We took this as a sign that she was relaxing and becoming more trustful. She smiled a bit more, too.

But those days of well-being were short-lived.

Two weeks after the second embolization, Katie felt severe throbbing pain over her posterior left calf, and the duskiness of her left great toe suddenly progressed to severe cyanosis. Her other toes also started getting dusky.

Her radiologist hoped that the poor circulation could be improved with I.V. medications. Unfortunately, her condition steadily grew worse. Her circulatory changes were caused by something called the "steal phenomenon." After her second embolization, the branch of the AVM to the lower leg had lost its nutrition from above. To compensate, arterial feeders then started "stealing" circulation from the normal vascular system of the foot, causing progressive color and temperature changes.

Katie's toes became gangrenous, and she had to be told. As you know, gangrene can horrify anyone, and we needed to soften the impact. The doctors explained that if her toes remained dry and uninfected, no surgery would have to be done. But if infection developed, the toes would have to be removed. Katie was plainly scared.

That evening, I talked to her about what her doctors had told her. She wanted her leg to be saved, she said. Its horrible appearance apparently made no difference to her. From groin to toe, it was swollen twice the size of her other leg. The thigh was warm and pink, but marked with prominent vessels, and you could actually feel a thrill from the AVM with your hand. The lower leg was ischemic and cyanotic, with a rapidly worsening sore under the heel and new ulcers developing on the back of the calf—further evidence of the steal of blood by the AVM. Looking at her leg every day, I realized that amputation might be necessary. The task now was to help her admit the same possibility.

Gingerly, I talked to her about all this. She expressed great sorrow and fear about losing her foot. Like most 13-year-olds, she worried more about what others might think and say than about how she would live. But even without toes, she knew she would still be able to perform on the parallel bars, although she couldn't conceive of what her life would be like if her leg were amputated. "I wouldn't be me," she said.

Her toes got blacker during the next few weeks, and a third embolization provided no improve-

ment. Her doctors decided to debride the leg ulcers and, at the same time, perform a distal metatarsal amputation. Although she didn't want to lose even a part of her foot, at least she understood that it wouldn't heal itself and suddenly become normal again. That meant she had certainly altered some of her expectations.

Her surgery went well and she adjusted easily to the dressing changes, which had to be done four times a day. An infection developed, though, and despite 3 weeks of antibiotic therapy, the neurovascular condition of her leg remained poor and the grafts didn't heal. Her doctors then decided that a definitive amputation was the only option.

She would have nothing to do with that option. She wanted her left leg too much. She said it was still useful and that she could prove it to all of us by working extra hard in physical therapy. "I won't give up my leg," she told her doctor.

The strength of that determination was soon tested. One day while she was on the parallel bars, her left leg began hemorrhaging and only a bulky pressure dressing could stop the bleeding. The experience caused her the worst pain she'd ever felt. An I.V. morphine drip was titrated to give her some relief. Afterward, she had the willpower to tell me that, despite all the bleeding, she still did *not* need more surgery.

But time was growing short. If the amputation wasn't performed—and soon—Katie would die from septicemia.

During the next 2 weeks, our goal was to improve her nutritional status so she could withstand surgery. But just as important, we had to guide her toward accepting the benefits of that operation. She refused to sign the operative consent, and her parents would only permit the amputation if she agreed to it first.

But she wouldn't. She thought that amputation meant an end to her life. She'd be considered unattractive. People wouldn't like her. And she'd have to give up gymnastics forever.

To convince her that she was wrong, we asked Susan, a 20-year-old amputee, to talk to Katie. We wanted Katie to understand that she could lead a normal—and active—life after losing a leg. Susan, who ice-skated and hiked for recreation, visited with her for nearly an hour, and although the 13-year-old didn't ask many questions, she sure listened. Afterward, she told me she thought Susan was brave. We made certain Katie understood that *she* was just as brave. Two days later, Katie and her parents finally agreed to the amputation.

After talking to Susan, she realized that the diseased leg was *not* her whole life—which is how she'd been regarding it for the past year. Her life was more than just her leg. She now understood that if its condition worsened, her leg would actually deprive her of her life.

Katie realized she had something else going for her. The same strength of will that had guided her through the last 8 months of pain and anxiety in the hospital could help her live a normal, active life, even if she had only one leg. With that decision, she took her first step from being a little girl to becoming a young woman.

During an 8½-hour operation, doctors performed a hip disarticulation. Because she lost nearly 20 pints (9.4 liters) of blood and had a history of complications, her immediate prognosis was guarded. But 5 hours later, she was awake and responsive. She was given I.V. morphine for pain, and we made sure she understood she would be able to talk the following day, after the endotracheal tube was removed.

Katie's first question was to me: "Is my leg really gone, Lauren?" Her second was, "Am I awful looking?" I told her she was prettier than ever. And she really was. In only a few hours, her face had undergone a dramatic change. Severe and tense before surgery, it now seemed gentle and relaxed. Psychologically, it was as if she had finally put down the terrible, heavy weight she'd been carrying for the past year.

During the next few days, her spirits brightened and she was transferred out of the intensive care unit after 6 days. She looked at her wounds during dressing changes, which I took as a sign that she had accepted her surgery. Her will to recover was almost incredible. It was as if by losing her diseased leg, she could finally start living again. Ten days after surgery, she sat up in a wheelchair and soon after walked with crutches.

Within 2 months of discharge, she was fitted with a prosthesis. That fall, she went back to school. She now works out on the parallel bars and, although she didn't make her school's gymnastics team, she's looking forward to helping coach the other kids. Also, she has her first "real" boyfriend. In other words, Katie Richards has become the typical teenager she wanted so desperately to be.

Caring for Katie showed us how much a patient's expectations play in recovery. When her expectations were unrealistically high, her progress was slow and agonizing. But once she learned to keep her options open, she could conquer her fear of surgery. With new hope, Katie can now look forward to taking her first steps toward adulthood.

Emma Needed More than Standard Teaching

MARJORIE HURLEY, RN, BSN
ANNE MEYER-RUPPEL, RN, BA
EVELYN EVANS, RN, BSN

We all know patient teaching helps prevent post-surgical complications and speed recovery. But for patients facing radical, mutilating surgery, a standard teaching plan isn't enough. They need a personal strategy to help them adjust to their altered body image.

Emma O'Brien, a 70-year-old childless widow, was one of those patients. Because of invasive vulvar cancer, she had a vulvectomy with bilateral lymph node dissection—a traumatizing and painful ordeal. Emma coped with her loss of self-esteem by denying her condition, which created serious problems when we tried to teach her self-care skills.

On our oncology unit, we choose our primary care patients, and at admission, we orient them to the unit. Besides helping the patients relax, these informal, introductory sessions give us a chance to find out how well they understand their illnesses. Each patient's level of awareness determines how much teaching we'll need to do.

With Emma, our work was really cut out for us. When one of us asked why she thought she was in the hospital, she casually replied, "I'm here for a checkup. Don't *you* know that?" What we knew was that she was scheduled for a series of tests for vulvar cancer and not for a simple checkup, as she believed. When we tried to explain the difference, her pale blue eyes flitted from side to side as if she had a hard time thinking about what we were saying.

After a short while, it became apparent that she didn't want to think about her upcoming tests at all. When we told her we'd be happy to answer any questions she might have about them, she paused for a moment before asking, "Do you think I'll be home for dinner tonight?" Then she gave us a toothy grin. We glanced at each other before explaining the tests would take about 3 days.

She looked surprised...*genuinely surprised.* "But I play bingo every Tuesday after dinner," she said. We told her she'd have to stay in the hospital until her tests were finished. And again she looked surprised. "My friends are going to miss me tonight," she said somewhat crossly. For Emma, her friends were a main source of emotional support.

And Emma needed all the emotional support she could get, especially after her test results came in. A colposcopic examination pinpointed a vulvar lesion, which the biopsy showed to be malignant. To make matters worse, 4 of the 12 pelvic lymph nodes on her right side tested positive. Since her cancer was so extensive, a radical vulvectomy requiring deep bilateral dissection of superficial and deep inguinal lymph nodes was necessary. The urethra and vagina would also be resected, leaving an open perineal wound for 2 to 3 months. The cancer center's policy is to reconstruct the vaginas of only sexually active women, so Emma wouldn't be a candidate for follow-up surgery.

As you can well understand, a radical vulvectomy is emotionally devastating. Like a mastectomy, this sexually mutilating operation shatters a woman's self-image, and some patients can't ever put the pieces back together again. As their self-esteem fades, so does their desire to do things for themselves. They become apathetic and depressed. We wanted to do everything we could to stop that from happening to Emma.

On our unit, we have a standardized care plan for vulvectomy patients. But no standardized care plan could possibly address Emma's complicated emotional needs. We'd have to do that ourselves with personal attention, reassurance—and honesty.

So, as soon as her doctors told her she'd been scheduled for a vulvectomy, we made sure we spent a lot of time with Emma. We explained that the surgery is safe and effective, and that afterward, she'd be able to live a fairly active life.

Then to give her a clear idea of what lay ahead, we showed her the preoperative teaching book we'd designed especially for vulvectomy patients. This book has been an invaluable aid in helping patients understand this frightening surgery. Inside was a series of photographs showing each stage of surgery.

As we turned the pages and carefully explained each picture, we watched Emma's face. She'd said very little since the doctors told her she needed surgery. But pointing to a picture of a patient irrigating her wound with a peri bottle, she finally blurted out exactly what was on her mind. "That looks god-awful," she said hoarsely, barely concealing her revulsion. "Will it always be so ugly?" We explained that with good wound healing, her body would eventually look quite normal. After we told her that, she seemed to relax a little, and

we thought she was starting to accept the idea of her vulvectomy.

But any progress we thought we'd made swiftly evaporated. Even the night before surgery, Emma was still clinging to a tattered thread of hope. "Well, maybe I won't need surgery after all," she sighed deeply. When she switched off her bedside table lamp, it seemed as though she was turning off our efforts at helping her.

Back from the operating room, Emma appeared withdrawn and sullen. We knew a war of emotions had been going on inside her—now the battle was really raging. That's why our postoperative teaching was different from our preoperative teaching. She didn't need long, involved explanations like before. Now she needed simple, direct answers to her questions. But as before, Emma didn't ask many questions at first. She told us she was in too much pain.

So we tried to make her as comfortable as possible. To relieve the tension on her incision and increase circulation, we placed a pillow between her knees. Then we gave her 100 mg of meperidine (pethidine, Demerol, Pethoid) intramuscularly (I.M.), p.r.n., and 75 mg of hydroxyzine HCl (Vistaril) I.M. every 3 to 4 hours. Prompt removal of her soiled dressings, adequate ventilation, and deodorant sprays made her room more pleasant.

To prevent infection, we gently scrubbed her wound with a detergent soap solution six times each day, encouraging her to watch us closely as we demonstrated the proper technique. We also placed her in a sitz bath for 10 to 20 minutes each day to enhance circulation. To promote healing, we exposed her wound to the air as often as possible, using a hair dryer on the lowest setting to keep the wound area dry.

A few days after the patient's surgery, we like to encourage her to try to do her own wound care. We want her to start confronting the reality of her body changes, which is vital for recovery. For most of our patients, it's not an easy step to take. And Emma was no exception. Once afraid of surgery, she now was too afraid to even look at her wound.

After filling the peri bottle, we'd hand it to her. Then, with her eyes averted, she'd make a few motions in the general vicinity of her perineum, mostly squirting her legs and buttocks, and quickly hand the bottle back. "I'm done now," she'd whisper. It was as if by ignoring her wound, she thought she could make it disappear.

And you know what? She *did* go to some rather creative extremes to ignore it. "The night nurse said I could wait until later for my irrigations," she lied to the afternoon nurse. She even began objecting to taking her daily sitz baths. More than once, she said, "The morning nurse said I don't need a bath today." For a while, her care really got confusing, so we scheduled frequent conferences and wrote clear, legible notes on Emma's Kardex. That helped us. But we knew all the notes in the world wouldn't help change her attitude.

On her third postsurgical day, we asked her if she'd like to try to walk. Because she'd suffered a temporary paralysis of her right leg from her lymph dissection, we'd ordered a walker for her. Surprisingly, she agreed without a word of protest.

We soon found out why. Emma was something of a social butterfly. She loved talking to people, and whenever she met someone on her short walks, she stopped to chat for a few minutes. Fascinated, we watched her. Whenever her friends visited, her face lit up. She became almost *charming*. But the moment she was back alone in her private room, she became surly and uncooperative, showing us how much she liked to be out on her own.

That's when we decided to motivate Emma by letting her make out her own daily schedule. Since she wouldn't cooperate with us when we wanted her to, maybe she would when *she* wanted to. "You mean I get to boss *you* around," she said, obviously intrigued.

Emma didn't hesitate a moment. Right away, she set the time of day when it was most convenient for her to eat, sleep, and have snacks. Then, she chose the best times to have her sitz bath. Finally, she decided she'd take her walks during visiting hours when socializing was easiest.

Once again, we modified our basic teaching plan to address her special needs. To make her feel more independent, for instance, we gave her a few practical tips to make everyday activities a little easier. We taught her how to squat and sit back slightly when urinating to avoid wetting her legs or the floor. We also explained how a low-residue diet would help her avoid straining while defecating and ease her discomfort.

After a week, she started making some progress. Despite all of our teaching, though, she still wouldn't irrigate her own wound. We had to come up with another plan—and *fast*.

To make it easier for her, we brought in a small hand mirror with a long handle. By holding the mirror with one hand, Emma could hold the peri bottle with her other hand. Of course, for our technique to work, she'd have to actually *look* into the mirror.

Even that was a struggle. We helped her by drawing attention to her wound—but in a very positive way. "Oh, look," we'd say to each other so she could hear us. "Emma's incision is healing really nicely." Despite our efforts, though, she continued to do her irrigations carelessly.

Up until this point, we'd been filling her peri bottles for her, but after a few more days, we taught her how to fill them herself. Every now and then, we noticed her giving the wound what might be called an *extended* glance. So to encourage her even more, we gently held her legs apart to expose the perineum while she cleansed herself. Gradually, she began to slow down her motions and do a more thorough job.

That's when we realized how important it had been to Emma that all along we'd accepted her changed appearance. By doing that, we enabled her to accept it herself.

During the next few days, we noticed a dramatic improvement in her attitude. A fast learner when she wanted to be, she was not only cleansing her wound correctly by the end of the week, but she was also doing her own wound packing.

Discharged 2 weeks later, Emma took care of herself with the help of a home health-care nurse. We knew that her adjustment would be gradual and take more than just a few weeks. That's important to remember when you're caring for a patient with an altered body image.

And it's also important to remember something else. A patient-teaching plan is like a road map. A definite plan, yes—but one with many options. Believe us: When your patient's facing the trauma of radical surgery—and especially a revision of body image—she'll really appreciate those options.

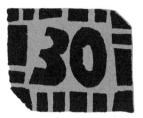

Mark's Wounds Were More than Physical

ELAINE A. TRAMPOSCH, RN, BSN

A patient's invisible wounds are often the hardest to treat. When Mark Spencer, 25, was admitted to our plastic surgery unit, he had glaring physical injuries—and some very well-hidden emotional ones.

Mark was transferred to us after 6 weeks in the intensive care unit. An auto accident had caused a major loss of skin from his left forearm and elbow, and had left the right side of his face severely disfigured. He'd lost his right ear and eye and most of the skin on that side of his head. He also had a fractured mandible and leakage of cerebrospinal fluid from the avulsed dura mater. Miraculously, though, he had no brain damage.

Just before transferring to our unit, Mark had been weaned from the ventilator, and the spinal catheter had been removed. But he still had a tracheostomy, and his jaws were wired shut.

For 6 weeks Mark had struggled to stay alive, and he'd won. Now we had to prepare him physically and emotionally for the painful ordeal that lay ahead.

From the beginning, Mark's physical care was overwhelming. At first, we checked on him every half hour, monitored his vital signs every hour, and suctioned him through his tracheostomy every 2 hours. Since his spinal catheter had been removed just before he came to our unit, we were concerned about spinal fluid leaking from the catheter site and increased intracranial pressure. So we performed hourly neurologic checks, testing Mark's pupillary response to light and asking him to move his extremities and squeeze our hands. We also tested the drainage from his head wound for cerebrospinal fluid. We had to turn him every 2 hours, keeping him off his right side. We also irrigated his left elbow every 2 hours and cleaned his head wound every 4 hours. This last procedure was probably the most painful.

Throughout his physical care, Mark seemed quiet and withdrawn—almost stoic. He'd wince in pain only when we removed his bandages, and occasionally, when the pain was especially severe, he'd raise a shaky arm to signal that he wanted to rest for a while. But he never tried to prevent us from doing his wound care, and more often than not he'd simply turn his head away when we entered his room.

During those first days, we were so preoccupied with Mark's physical care that we didn't pay much attention to his withdrawal behavior. With jaws wired shut and a tracheostomy, he couldn't speak, but he *could've* nodded yes or no. Instead, he just shrugged his shoulders whenever we asked him a question.

Thinking that Mark might be happier *writing* his thoughts, we gave him a pencil and paper. But writing was a terrible chore for him. First of all, he was right-handed and had trouble focusing on the paper with his left eye. Then he had to write with his bandaged left arm because his right arm was immobilized by a central venous line and an armboard. So naturally, we worried that Mark might not convey problems to us if any arose.

But despite his noncommunicativeness, Mark was basically cooperative. He only complained when he needed pain medication or, occasionally, when we had to suction him. Before the week was up, though, I got my first indication that underneath Mark's silent stoicism lay a whole network of explosive feelings and fears.

One day I was preparing to help him with his morning care, when he asked for his paper and pencil and wrote that he could do the care himself. I agreed to let him try, glad that he seemed so motivated. I put a basin, facecloth, towel, and soap on his overbed tray and told him I'd be back in a few minutes, if he needed help.

When I returned, Mark was sitting straight up in bed, looking in the fold-up mirror on the tray. Tears were streaming down his face. I gently questioned him, and he admitted with a shake of his head that he hadn't seen his facial injuries before. Then he fiercely pounded his right fist into the bed—over and over.

Holding his hand, I apologized for having left him alone, explaining that I thought he'd already seen his injuries. But he reached for his paper and wrote that he wanted to be alone. Before I left, I told him if he felt like talking later, I'd be there to listen.

But I had the sinking feeling that Mark would never mention the incident again. I was only just beginning to understand the psychological problems this young man was facing.

Mark had once been a handsome, active man. He was married, had a 2-year-old son, and owned

a construction business. Now he was severely disfigured, confined to a hospital bed, and was being cared for by a group of women just about his own age. I began to see that much of Mark's reticence was based on pride—he wanted to be regarded as a *normal* man. Also, he was probably embarrassed because we had to do so many things for him, yet he cooperated because he was anxious to regain control and dignity in his life.

So we added some important goals to our care plan. We had to help Mark assume as much control as possible, help him feel like a man and a vital part of his family again, and encourage him to feel comfortable enough with us to express his feelings more openly. We began by letting him take an active part in his care.

Because Mark's daily care was so extensive, we had to adhere to a detailed care plan—otherwise, we'd never get our work done and Mark would never get any sleep. Still, we tried to make the plan as flexible as possible to give Mark some say in his daily activities. For example, we told him what time we'd take his vital signs and what time

 Mark had once been a handsome, active man. Now he was severely disfigured, confined to a hospital bed, and was being cared for by a group of women just about his own age.

we'd turn him. Then based on our schedule, he could decide when he wanted to be washed, helped out of bed, or allowed to sleep.

We also tried to give Mark some privacy in his personal care, although admittedly, this was often impossible. We knew he was embarrassed that we had to help him on and off the bedpan. And sometimes we *were* like mother hens, fussing over him, positioning him, lubricating his back— this embarrassed him, too. So Mark started letting us know when we were fussing too much by making little clicking sounds to express his annoyance. Then, even though we couldn't avoid doing almost everything for him, we'd try to finish his care as unobtrusively as possible and give him some time alone.

Whenever we could, we found ways to let Mark participate in his care. One concern in preparing Mark for surgery was improving his nutritional status. He'd lost 60 pounds since his accident and couldn't eat by mouth when he first came to us. When continuing I.V. hydration became difficult, we asked Mark if he'd like to try some fluids, and he agreed. We started with water the first day, and then switched to a high-carbohydrate drink. Soon Mark was taking small, frequent amounts of juice, broth, Isocal, and milk shakes through a straw. He plotted his slow, steady weight gain by keeping his own intake and output records and by jotting down his daily weight.

Another way he helped was by keeping track of his injection sites. Mark received meperidine (pethidine, Demerol, Pethoid) and hydroxyzine (Vistaril, Atarax) intramuscularly a half hour before each wound care session. This amounted to six injections a day, so we had to rotate sites. Mark always knew just where each injection should be given.

Despite these small breakthroughs, Mark still wasn't communicating much; although we made some progress when we taught him to speak by plugging his tracheostomy opening. At first, we had trouble understanding him, but with practice on both sides we began communicating better. Mark seemed happy about this and told us that using the pad and pencil had just been too much trouble. He began initiating conversations with us—usually about neutral subjects like television programs. And occasionally he'd ask questions about his surgery. We tried getting him to talk about his family and any worries he might have, but he refused to discuss anything personal.

Finally, we approached his family ourselves. Both his mother and his wife (a nurse) were frequent visitors, and they seemed to be handling the situation well. Mark's wife told me that Mark had always been a private person, so she didn't feel that his reticence was anything unusual. But then, blushing slightly, she admitted that she hadn't really encouraged Mark to discuss his problems.

"Being a nurse doesn't make things any easier when the patient's your husband," she said.

With our encouragement, Mrs. Spencer finally got Mark to discuss his worries, and he told her he was most concerned about how their son, Robert, would react when he saw Mark's facial injuries.

We tried to get Mark to discuss his concerns with us, too, but he continued to retreat when it came to talking about his feelings. Whenever we mentioned his son, though, he perked up noticeably. So as soon as the doctors felt that Mark's head wound was free of infection, we got special permission to let Robert visit.

Before the visit, we spent many sessions with Mark, discussing Robert's possible reactions. We reminded Mark that when Robert saw him covered with bandages, he might be overwhelmed. Robert might feel angry with Mark for staying away so long, or he might not even recognize him at first.

Mark admitted there were risks involved but remained strong in his desire to see his son. And the day Mark's wife brought Robert in was probably the most emotional of Mark's hospital stay. Robert went right to his father and seemed to accept the explanation that "daddy has a 'boo-boo' and needs bandages."

Afterward, Mark turned to us and whispered, "You don't know how good I feel knowing I'm not a stranger to my boy."

It was probably the most heartfelt thing he'd ever said to us. We frequently referred to this episode to remind Mark that his inner qualities were still the same, and his family would always know this.

In trying to draw Mark out, we learned that he loved to talk about his work. He enthusiastically described the houses he'd built and often showed us pictures of them. So he was genuinely excited when the doctor told him he'd be able to return to work one day.

Although Mark never did talk openly to us about his fears concerning his physical appearance, he did ask about his upcoming surgery: when and how it would be done, and what he would look like afterward.

"Will I look good?" he always asked, but he'd clam up if we tried to pursue his feelings about this.

We tried to be consistent in our answers to Mark and encourage him without giving him false hope. His doctors explained the stages necessary to reconstruct his head, zygomatic arch, and jaw, and to fit him with an ear and eye prosthesis. We emphasized that the bone graft would restore the contour of his face, and the prosthetic ear and eye would enhance his appearance greatly. But we admitted that it was too early to predict the results.

We thought that talking to another patient who'd gone through facial surgery might help Mark. So one day, as I was changing his dressing, I brought up the subject. I explained that we had another patient in his 20s, Tom, who had similar injuries.

"His surgery is almost finished and he really looks good," I said.

Mark seemed interested and asked a few questions about Tom and his surgery. I asked if he'd like to arrange a meeting. Mark hesitated, then agreed.

Tom visited Mark the next day and talked unselfconsciously about his injuries and surgery. He explained to Mark how the doctors had restored his cheekbones with an iliac bone graft. Mark asked about the pain after surgery, and Tom replied honestly—there *was* a lot of pain, but it decreased after about 2 days.

They didn't speak long, but Tom promised to visit Mark again. Later, Mark asked if he would look as good as Tom. I reminded him that it was too early to predict the results, but emphasized the positive aspects of the surgery.

Shortly afterward, the doctors began grafting Mark's wound and applying pigskin to the remaining areas to protect them until they could be grafted. We taught Mark's wife to apply the pigskin, so for the first time in 3 months, Mark could go home for a while.

When Mark returned for suturing of an abdominal flap to his forearm, he'd gained about 20 pounds and looked much healthier and happier.

But looks can be deceiving. Unfortunately, Mark had severe postoperative pain, and then the abdominal flap became cyanotic. He became more withdrawn than before—actually sullen—and he stopped cooperating with us. He accused us of refusing to answer his call light or give his pain medication on time, and told us we were mean and the doctors were incompetent. Finally, he threatened to sign himself out of the hospital.

We realized then that a psychiatric consultation was long overdue. We asked a psychiatrist to visit Mark, and the psychiatrist convinced him not to leave the hospital. He visited Mark regularly throughout the rest of his hospitalization, and after discharge, Mark continued to get psychiatric help.

Mark had always been so cooperative and uncomplaining we'd assumed he was adjusting on his own. But we must remember that extremes in behavior can signal denial—very quiet or cooperative as well as very cheerful or optimistic patients may only *seem* to be coping with their illnesses or injuries.

As for Mark, reconstructing his face would take 2 or 3 more years and numerous trips to the hospital. And although we might have called for psychiatric help sooner, I think we did help lay the groundwork for Mark's recovery. True, we didn't work any miracles, and the results of our efforts were sometimes hard to see. But that's often the case when you're dealing with a patient's feelings. Those invisible wounds need the gentlest touch, and the healing can be painfully slow.

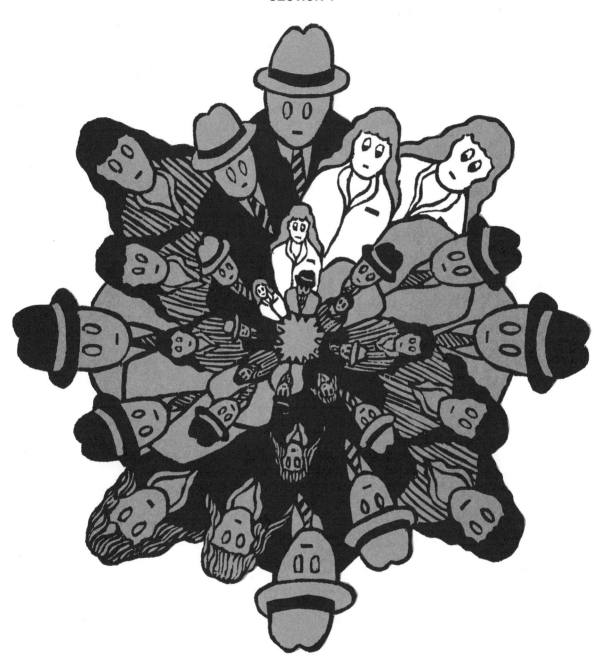

PATIENTS WITH PROBLEM FAMILIES

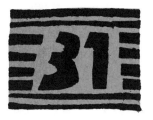

For Billy, Home Is Where the Hurt Is

RUTH ANN BURNS, RN, MSN

When they give their best to an effort, most people expect to succeed—that seems only fair. We nurses are no exception; we'd like all our case histories to turn into success stories. But sometimes when we have to settle for less, we discover we've gained more than we realize.

That's what happened when we tried to help Billy, a young patient with a daunting array of problems, including feuding parents.

Tall and thin, with intense dark eyes, 16-year-old Billy Boyce had the look of a young Edgar Allan Poe. Once he opened his mouth, though, those weren't sonnets he was spouting; they were obscenities that would fluster a first mate.

This uncontrolled language occurs in about 60% of patients who have Tourette's syndrome, Billy's diagnosis when admitted to the psychiatric unit where I used to work. The syndrome, which is also characterized by rapid, repetitive movements (tics) and multiple verbal tics, can appear in children as young as 2 but rarely appears in children older than 13. In that, Billy's case was atypical.

His stay on our unit was unexpectedly brief. His mother had him discharged within a week. As she explained, "He's going to go to a Tourette's clinic in a few weeks. Besides, I want my baby home with me."

While home, Mrs. Boyce's "baby" deliberately plunged his right hand into a pot of scalding hot coffee. After his second-degree burns were treated, he was readmitted to our unit.

No foul talk this time. Scarcely any talk at all. Billy was withdrawn, unwilling to make eye contact, virtually mute. Strangely, he could ask for strawberry milk shakes clearly; otherwise, he only grunted. His hand movements were ritualistic. He was constantly rubbing his fingers together, especially those of his burned hand. Until we took him into the bathroom, that is. Then he tried to put his burned hand under hot water. Luckily, we stopped him.

Once Billy's burns had begun to heal, his mother had him discharged again. "He's better off with me," she said.

About 1 month later, Billy returned to us. Tourette's syndrome had been ruled out. This time his diagnosis was mixed specific developmental disorder with infantile autism, residual state. Billy's history indicated his language development was somewhat delayed, and he had considerable trouble learning to write.

Infantile autism, which develops before 30 months of age, usually involves lack of response to others, grossly deficient language development, and bizarre responses to environment. A diagnosis of infantile autism, residual state, means that although not all of these symptoms are present, the child is awkward socially and has trouble communicating. That seemed to describe Billy.

Because the neurologist had suspected a disturbance in sensory integration, Billy was tested by our occupational therapy department. Trouble in planning and performing skilled or nonhabitual tasks and clumsiness in motor activity characterize this disorder.

The child with a sensory integration problem may also have poor verbal skills and eye control. He has trouble dressing, learning to write, and constructing things because his brain can't perceive and integrate incoming stimuli. Distorted body image, poor self-concept, unusual movements or behavior, poor posture, and generally slow reflexes can result from the primary problem.

Billy did display many of these symptoms. He had delayed reflexive responses and couldn't distinguish various tactile sensations; his aversion to showers and water indicated tactile defensiveness.

He also seemed to show right-sided neglect. When we asked Billy to trace a figure in the air, he could cross the midline of his body. But when we asked him to place his right hand on his left ear, he turned his head to the right, indicating a reluctance to cross the body midline.

Billy's neurologist had ruled out organic causes for his behavior. Billy's psychiatrist, suspecting an endogenous affective disorder, requested a dexamethasone suppression test. The test results were positive, and a diagnosis of affective disorder, bipolar, mixed, was added to the growing list. The psychiatrist started Billy on a regimen of lithium carbonate for endogenous affective disorder.

As you can imagine, considering his many diagnoses, caring for Billy was challenging. Our best approach, we thought, was a multidisciplinary effort involving behavior modification, lithium, and family therapy.

Step one was to identify behaviors Billy could change. Step two was to come up with some positive reinforcers to encourage desirable behaviors. We tried to avoid negative reinforcement as much as possible.

Once we explained the program to Billy, he quickly agreed to some of our requests. He stopped trying to run away; he also stopped masturbating in public. Yet change came less readily in other areas.

When Billy's mother or father came to visit, for example, Billy played the clock as skillfully as a basketball team with a slim lead. He'd stand across the lounge from his visitor, continually change seats, or run down the hallway. But as the visitor began to leave at the end of visiting hours, Billy would clutch the visitor's legs and beg him to stay.

We began to play the clock, too, by establishing a new rule: Once a visitor arrived on the unit, Billy had to interact with him within 5 minutes. No contact within 5 minutes meant he really didn't want to see the visitor; we'd ask the visitor to leave. Strictly enforcing this rule helped control Billy's manipulation and eased his visitors' frustration.

Billy also tried to manipulate the staff, especially at mealtimes. He'd sit for more than an hour, just poking at his food like a suspicious health inspector. So we limited each meal to a half hour. Billy ate very little the first 3 days.

On the fourth day, he began to eat—but his dessert first. Our countermove was to take it away from his tray until he ate his entrée. Eventually his mealtime habits improved, so we didn't have to remove his dessert.

Billy's sensory problems caused the most difficult behavior problems. He hated taking showers, for instance. The occupational therapist on the team suggested that we let Billy take baths since they'd threaten his tactile sense less. At first, Billy would step in and out of the tub several times during the bath, or he'd refuse to get out of the tub once his bath was over. Within a few weeks, however, he seemed to enjoy his baths.

Washing Billy's hair was a "hair-raising" experience for all concerned. Billy would shriek and struggle whenever we poured water over his head. To decrease his sensory stimulation, we'd use a small cup for rinsing. Over time, we were able to increase the size of the container. Billy's struggling stopped, but we were never able to get him to wash his hair himself. Nor were we ever able to get him to brush his teeth.

But our success with most of the activities of daily living, besides improving Billy's basic hygiene, also helped minimize some of his sensory integration problems. For example, to bathe or dress, Billy had to cross the midline of the body. We'd place a washcloth in his right hand, asking him to wash the left side of his body. Or we'd tell him to button his left shirt cuff while dressing. Little by little he performed these maneuvers more easily.

Before Billy's behavior had become so progressively disruptive, he'd been on the track team at his school. So we added jogging to his behavior modification program to provide exercise and fresh air. He enjoyed this activity so much that he'd glow even before the jogging.

As Billy's interaction with the staff improved, we learned he had the teenage boy's typical passion for sports. Several of the male staff members began to play a game they called "sports trivia" with him. Who was the "Iron Man" of baseball? Billy knew.

On the whole, Billy's behavior modification program worked quite well. Adding lithium to Billy's medical regimen seemed to increase his ability to follow the program. He gradually could perform more and more complex tasks—and earned more and more stars.

The stars were almost a reward in and of themselves. However, the program did involve exchanging the stars for privileges. Billy consistently parlayed his stars into passes home; this was probably the worst aspect of our plan.

For Billy, home is where the hurt is.

According to the history Billy's mother gave to the family therapist, her marriage had been falling apart for 17 of its 17 years. In fact, she'd become pregnant with Billy during the honeymoon, and when her husband wanted her to get an abortion, she'd refused.

The brief honeymoon over, the long war had begun. Over the years, the parents repeatedly threw insults—and punches—at each other in front of the boy. Not the best home life for any child, let alone one with Billy's problems.

The Boyces consistently "triangled" Billy. In this triangle, Mrs. Boyce and Billy were the close twosome; Mr. Boyce, the outsider. Mrs. Boyce was overly involved with Billy and his illness. Mr. Boyce, on the other hand, was cold and emotionally detached from both mother and son. Still, he was intensely involved in the situation and refused to consider divorce despite continuous marital strife.

After the family therapist had several unproductive sessions with the Boyces, the team decided the therapist should align with Billy, provide feedback about his position in the family, and try to extricate him from the "triangle." That plan was somewhat successful.

For example, when both parents tried to get the therapist to take sides, she said she could feel them pulling her in opposite directions. She added, "If I feel I'm being pulled, surely Billy must have frequently felt the same way." A shy smile from Billy showed she was right.

Unfortunately, dynamic family therapy appeared impossible for the Boyces. Billy's problems and the family situation dictated separation from the parents and, after a 4-month stay with us, Billy was transferred to the only facility in the state that offered a sensory integration program. That facility was some 400 miles away, but the distance just might allow Billy some growing space.

When Billy left, many of us felt let down. Sure, he had improved because of our care. But the regret remained—if only we could have helped him more. He had such a long road ahead of him.

Yet we'd gotten some unexpected benefits from our experience with Billy. We had a better appreciation and more respect for the other disciplines on our unit. We knew we all gave our very best; we gained a pride in ourselves and our colleagues as professionals.

From what we'd learned, we could work to make our best better for our next patient—our next chance at being part of a success story.

Mrs. Ladley Thought She Could Care for Her Husband Better than We Could

SHARON PORTER, RN, MSN, CCRN

We've heard a lot lately about being the "patient's advocate," and no one can deny that patients *do* need our support. But sometimes we can get so carried away with our supportive role that we don't want anyone else interfering—even the patient's family.

Mr. Ladley was so passive and withdrawn, we didn't know what to do for him. So Mrs. Ladley *told* us—in no uncertain terms. She was convinced that she could care for her husband better than we could, and she resented *our* interference as much as we resented *hers.* Before we could help Mr. Ladley, we had to make Mrs. Ladley our ally. But how?

Sixty-eight-year-old Mr. Ladley had had a thoracotomy to remove a malignant tumor from his chest. Because of complications, he'd spent a month in the intensive care unit before being transferred to the medical/surgical unit. In spite of hyperalimentation therapy, he was malnourished and emaciated. And as if his list of problems wasn't long enough, he'd been a paraplegic for 35 years.

We started off on the wrong foot with Mrs. Ladley right away. Shortly after Mr. Ladley's trans-

fer, he developed a decubitus ulcer on his sacrum. Mrs. Ladley immediately filed a complaint with the director of nursing, and that's how I came into the picture. As a clinical nurse specialist in critical care, I was doing a study on using a skin barrier adhesive in decubitus treatment. The nursing supervisor thought Mr. Ladley would be a good patient to include in the study.

But she warned me that *Mrs.* Ladley would be a problem. The staff nurses reported that she seemed obsessed with every detail of her husband's illness and refused to leave his bedside. They put a cot in his room so she could spend nights with him—otherwise, she'd probably have slept in a chair.

"Don't even bother asking Mr. Ladley any questions," the supervisor said. "His wife does all his talking for him."

Needless to say, I wasn't looking forward to meeting Mrs. Ladley. If she was as difficult as she sounded, I hoped I could heal her husband's ulcer quickly.

But the first time I entered the room, I could see that the ulcer was the *least* of Mr. Ladley's problems. Mrs. Ladley was holding up her husband's sheet and pointing to his exposed sacral area while she lectured another nurse on decubitus care. Mr. Ladley just lay on his side, totally withdrawn.

The other nurse excused herself, a look of relief on her face, and I introduced myself to the Ladleys. Mrs. Ladley shook my hand vigorously, but Mr. Ladley never acknowledged me. So I tried one more time:

"How are you feeling today, Mr. Ladley?" I asked.

"He's *not good,* can't you see that?" Mrs. Ladley snapped.

Okay, I'll just concentrate on his physical care, I decided. I assessed the ulcer and then began explaining my treatment plan to Mrs. Ladley. She listened intently and asked several questions. Then she described her own care plan. Apparently she did almost everything for Mr. Ladley, including giving him an enema after breakfast, dressing him, and supervising his rest times. And besides being his full-time nurse, she helped him run the antique shop they owned.

I left that day with mixed emotions. No doubt about it. Mrs. Ladley *was* a difficult person. With her husband, she was overbearing and overprotective at the same time. But she obviously gave him good physical care—as good as any nurse—and I admired her for that. At the same time, I was appalled at the impersonal way she treated him—exposing him needlessly and discussing his problems as if he weren't even there. I wondered why Mr. Ladley allowed his wife to dominate him so.

After a week, I was making good progress healing the decubitus, but I was making no other kind of progress with the Ladleys. Mr. Ladley still wouldn't talk, so I started directing all my questions to Mrs. Ladley, who always answered anyway. But I felt guilty—now *I* was treating Mr. Ladley impersonally.

I wanted to talk to him alone, but Mrs. Ladley wouldn't take the hint. I didn't dare ask her to leave and risk destroying our already tenuous relationship.

One day, though, when she did leave the room for a few minutes, I quickly put my face level with Mr. Ladley's and stared straight into his eyes.

"Would you rather have me do your dressing changes some other time of day?" I asked, wanting him to know he had some say in the matter. After several minutes, he finally uttered one word: "No."

The nurses on the unit commented on how well Mr. Ladley's decubitus was healing and asked me about my treatment plan. But they seldom inquired

The staff nurses vented a great deal of anger at Mrs. Ladley— for criticizing them for the way they cared for her husband, when she herself treated him like a thing. "You know, she's just like the stereotype of a 'bad nurse,' " one nurse said. "She treats the illness and ignores the patient."

about my personal relationship with the Ladleys. The nurses had long since given up trying to communicate with Mr. Ladley, and from what they told me, they walked a tightrope with Mrs. Ladley, just as I did.

But I had an advantage over the other nurses— I had one uninterrupted hour a day to spend with the Ladleys, without any pressure from other patients. Consequently, I felt I understood the Ladley's problems better, that perhaps I had things in better perspective than the other nurses. So I asked the supervisor if we could hold a staff conference to discuss the Ladleys.

During the conference, the staff nurses vented a great deal of anger at Mrs. Ladley—for criticizing *them* for the way *they* cared for her husband, when she herself treated him like a "thing."

"You know, she's just like the stereotype of a

'bad nurse,'" one nurse said. "She treats the illness and ignores the patient."

I had to agree, yet I also had to point out, "We're caring for Mr. Ladley under the *best* conditions, and it's still not easy. Imagine what it's like for Mrs. Ladley at home."

By the end of the conference, we'd all begun coming to terms with our feelings. We agreed that without Mrs. Ladley, Mr. Ladley could never be discharged back home, and that regardless of whether we *liked* Mrs. Ladley, we needed *her* help as much as she needed *ours.*

During our conference, we also wrote a new care plan—not just for Mr. Ladley, but for Mrs. Ladley, too. Our goal: to prepare Mr. Ladley for discharge. Our chief consultant: Mrs. Ladley.

I explained the care plan to the Ladleys right away. Of course, Mr. Ladley showed no interest. But when I told Mrs. Ladley that she'd be responsible for much of her husband's care, she said righteously, "It's about time."

That day, I helped Mrs. Ladley do her husband's decubitus care. She caught on quickly and also made several suggestions about other aspects of his care. She told me which foods he liked best, that he enjoyed a glass of wine before dinner, and that he loved to watch football on TV. I incorporated all her suggestions into the care plan. When I left that day, I knew we could count on Mrs. Ladley to take over much of her husband's physical care.

We hoped that we could interest Mr. Ladley in eating again, thinking that if he felt better physically, he might feel less depressed. Even with hyperalimentation, he still wasn't gaining enough weight, so the dietitian helped us plan a 2,000 calorie/day menu that included the foods Mr. Ladley liked. Still he refused to eat, so Mrs. Ladley fed him and then recorded his daily food intake for the dietitian.

After a few days, Mr. Ladley *was* eating more, but he still wouldn't participate in his care in any way. We asked our social worker to visit the Ladleys and, although the social worker never got more than a one-word answer from Mr. Ladley, she did talk privately to Mrs. Ladley. She pointed out, as tactfully as she could, how Mrs. Ladley's habit of answering for her husband only added to his withdrawn state. But even though Mrs. Ladley listened

politely, she continued to do her husband's talking for him. Perhaps she simply couldn't break such a long-standing habit.

Almost in spite of himself, Mr. Ladley began getting physically stronger. The doctor gave us permission to get him into a wheelchair, and we asked the physical therapist to begin working with him.

For a while, we simply lifted Mr. Ladley into a chair three times a day. He reacted (or rather, *didn't* react) by staring at the opposite wall. But when we took him for a wheelchair ride to the pediatric unit, we thought we saw a flicker of interest in his eyes. The next day, we took him outside on the patio—the first time he'd been out in almost 2 months. And although he never spoke a word, the expression on his face spoke volumes—for the first time, he smiled.

Later that week, Mrs. Ladley took him to the hospital dining room for lunch. When they returned, she was elated. "I started to feed him,"

> *We agreed that without Mrs. Ladley, Mr. Ladley could never be discharged back home and that regardless of whether we liked Mrs. Ladley, we needed her help as much as she needed ours.*

she said, "and he told me he could feed himself. Then he *did.*"

At last Mr. Ladley was coming out of his shell. He still wouldn't talk if his wife was present, but if she was gone, he'd answer our questions. He seemed to enjoy his wheelchair rides and had begun to watch football games on TV. We made a point not to disturb him while he was watching a game, but we also made a point of asking him who was playing and what the score was. If Mrs.

Ladley was out of the room, he'd tell us.

We made an extra effort to compliment Mr. Ladley on his successes and encourage him to do more for himself. We also tried to keep our conversations as upbeat as possible, so he wouldn't become more depressed.

Then a week before his discharge, Mr. Ladley suddenly began vomiting all his food. An upper GI series showed an esophageal stricture, but the doctor didn't feel that Mr. Ladley was strong enough to tolerate another thoracotomy. So the doctor dilated the stricture twice a week, gradually increasing the size of the dilators. To our great relief, Mr. Ladley didn't sink into a deeper depression—maybe because we reassured him that Mrs. Ladley could learn to do the procedure at home.

We weren't prepared for what happened next. When the doctor told Mrs. Ladley he wanted to teach her to use the dilators, she burst into tears. "How much more can I be expected to do?" she sobbed.

We were shocked. Mrs. Ladley had never shown one sign of weakness before—she'd always exuded confidence and capability. For the first time, we realized how overwhelmed she really felt and how little we'd thought about her feelings. We'd been so busy encouraging Mr. Ladley that we'd hardly given Mrs. Ladley a word of encouragement.

After that, we made a point of spending some time alone with her every day. We told her how much we admired her for the care she'd given her husband—that his very survival was a tribute to her care. We complimented her on how quickly she'd learned each new procedure and also on how much she'd taught *us* about caring for a paraplegic at home.

That was the boost Mrs. Ladley needed. She began learning how to use the dilators, and when Mr. Ladley was discharged 2 weeks later, she'd mastered the technique.

Although we never saw the Ladleys again, we thought about them often. We'll never know how great a part we played in making their relationship a happier one, but we'd like to think that with our help, Mr. Ladley became a little more self-sufficient, and Mrs. Ladley, a little less overbearing.

But our experience with the Ladleys left us with more than just unanswered questions. We learned that to truly be the patient's advocate, sometimes we have to be his family's advocate, too—even if this means relinquishing some of our responsibility.

A Letter from Tommy

RANDI FULLER, RN, BSN
MARTHA PETERING, RN, MN

When your difficult patient is a tiny infant, your job can take on immense proportions. And when the infant has a physical abnormality that one of his parents can't accept, your job becomes harder still.

Tommy Sutton had a serious problem—hyaline membrane disease. But his mother had a problem, too—she didn't even want to see him, much less take part in his care. We knew we could make Tommy well enough to go home; but first, we had to be sure he had someone to go home *to*.

Tommy was born 2 weeks prematurely. The doctors at the community hospital diagnosed respiratory distress syndrome and immediately made plans to transfer him to an advanced care hospital 60 miles away.

Assigned to be Tommy's primary care nurse, I went along in the ambulance to pick him up. While the doctor examined him, I asked the nurses at the community hospital to fill me in.

They told me that the Suttons were in their early 30s and had two other children. Mrs. Sutton had worked in the hospital's central supply department and was now on maternity leave. *Good, she'll be familiar with hospital procedures and equipment,* I thought. *Teaching her to care for Tommy at home shouldn't be too hard.*

But then the nurses told me something that made my heart sink—Mrs. Sutton hadn't visited Tommy once since his birth. And when they tried to talk to her about him, her only question was, "Will he live?"

In evaluating Mrs. Sutton's reaction, I couldn't help but remember that early initial contact is the most important factor in establishing a positive maternal-child bond. Visual inspection and tactile exploration by the mother are particularly important if the infant's being transferred to a hospital far away from his parents. But Tommy'd been whisked away from his mother at birth, before she'd even had a chance to touch him; and now he was being whisked away again. And to make matters worse, for some reason—fear, perhaps, or guilt—Mrs. Sutton didn't even *want* to see her son.

Maybe she wouldn't have time to establish a bond with Tommy before his transfer, but at least I could make sure she saw him once.

I introduced myself to Mrs. Sutton, told her I'd

be Tommy's new primary care nurse, and explained that he'd probably be hospitalized for at least 2 months. When I told her I'd bring Tommy to her so she could say good-bye, her eyes opened wide in alarm. But before she could protest, I wheeled the incubator into her room.

"He's a perfectly lovely little boy, Mrs. Sutton," I said reassuringly. "He just needs some help from the ventilator to breathe. But as soon as he's gained a little weight and can breathe on his own, you can take him home."

Mrs. Sutton peeked cautiously into the incubator; and when she saw that Tommy looked normal, she seemed relieved. I urged her to touch him, and she touched his arm very tentatively. Then she settled back on the pillows as if to say, "I've had enough." I told her we'd take good care of her baby and that she could call us anytime and check on Tommy.

The doctors at our hospital diagnosed Tommy's problem as hyaline membrane disease. Besides mechanical ventilation, his medical care plan included intubation and an umbilical artery catheter to monitor blood gases and provide intravenous fluids.

Mrs. Sutton didn't call once during the first week. Mr. Sutton, however, visited three times. He'd sit by the incubator, staring at his son with mournful eyes. Occasionally, he'd poke a cautious hand through the porthole and stroke the baby's cheek. But when we asked if he'd like to hold Tommy, he looked scared to death and always said "no."

A week after his admission, Tommy began to have complications. He developed a tension pneumothorax and a pneumonomediastinum secondary to atelectasis, so the doctor inserted chest tubes. Then, just as these problems were under control, he began having inspiratory stridor and expiratory wheezing, and his PCO_2 level increased. He was fighting so hard for breath that he developed deep chest wall retractions. A bronchoscopy revealed subglottic stenosis, so the doctors did a tracheotomy.

As Tommy's problems increased, so did ours. Since only a few nurses in our unit had ever cared for a tracheotomized infant, we asked our clinical specialist in neonatology to give us pointers on how to care for him.

Three weeks passed. By now, we'd expected Mrs. Sutton to feel well enough to visit. But she never even called. I called her regularly, though, encouraging her to visit and reporting on Tommy's condition. I always stressed the baby's strong points—how much weight he'd gained, what good muscle tone he had, how cute he was. Then, I'd mention some of the things she'd need to learn before Tommy could go home—how to use the suctioning equipment, how to clean and change the inner cannula of the tracheostomy tube. "It sounds scary, I know, but really it isn't that hard," I'd tell her. "I could *never* learn that," she insisted, and seemed frankly horrified at the idea. I tried to build up her confidence, telling her we'd teach her everything she needed to know. But all the while, I wondered, *How can we teach her if she won't even visit?*

So I'd try another tactic—stressing the *patient's* strong points. "You've worked in a hospital, so you already know what the equipment looks like, Mrs. Sutton. I'm sure you won't have any trouble learning how to use it." But she'd always answer, "I could never learn how."

Mr. Sutton was depressed. He told us that his wife had used every excuse in the book for not visiting Tommy—she couldn't leave her other children; she didn't have a car; she didn't have any money for train fare because her maternity benefits hadn't started yet. We called our social service department, and they told us they had a special fund to cover transportation expenses for needy parents. So we made arrangements for Mrs. Sutton to come by train. She refused.

Tommy had been weaned from the ventilator for 2 weeks and was growing stronger every day. But Mrs. Sutton hadn't weakened one iota. Tommy would be well enough to go home in a month; but first, someone had to learn how to care for him. Teaching *Mr.* Sutton wasn't the answer. Mrs. Sutton had raised two other children and was surely better equipped to care for Tommy's needs.

We'd been sympathetic with Mrs. Sutton at first—accepting Tommy's illness wasn't easy. But now, after weeks of pleading and cajoling over the phone, we weren't sympathetic anymore. We were *desperate*.

But sometimes, the best ideas are born out of desperation. One day, when I was feeding Tommy, I realized he was more my baby than his moth-

Dear Mom and Dad,

Randi and I want to tell you a little about my tracheostomy tube, so you can start taking care of me. Here's our plan for teaching you my trach care so I can come home.

1. First you'll learn how to take out the inner cannula.

2. Next, you'll learn how to clean the inner cannula.

3. Then you'll practice doing my suctioning and chest physical therapy.

4. And last, you'll learn how to change my trach tube (my nurse will show you how).

Don't worry — I'll be as good as gold so it'll be easy. I can't wait to come home so please come soon.

Love,
Tommy

er's—simply because I'd held him and cared for him. I felt angry and almost reached for the phone to call Mrs. Sutton. Then I thought, anger's destructive, do something constructive. And that's when I thought of the letter—"written" by Tommy to his parents (see illustration).

Tommy's letter was the turning point for us and for the Suttons. The day Mrs. Sutton received the letter, she called me to say she accepted the hospital's offer to pay her train fare, and she'd come to visit the next day.

Our discharge teaching program had been ready for weeks, but we reviewed it one more time. With the clinical specialist's help, we'd become experts at giving tracheostomy care to infants.

Our goal was to make Mrs. Sutton an expert, too, and then, to help her teach Mr. Sutton. We set a 1 month limit for completing our discharge teaching; but if necessary, we were willing to spend a longer time, until the Suttons felt confident enough to take Tommy home.

We were so excited, we felt like decorating the nursery; but we decided to decorate Tommy, instead. One of the nurses had made him a hat and booties, and we dressed him in them, hoping that these small, personal touches might draw Mrs. Sutton's attention away from the tubes and equipment. Then we moved a rocker into an empty corner, so Mrs. Sutton would feel more at home when she held Tommy. While we waited for Mrs. Sutton to arrive, we felt jittery.

We needn't have worried—the first visit went beautifully. Sure, we had a few nervous moments, like when we showed Mrs. Sutton the tracheostomy, and she gasped and put her hand over her mouth. But we went slowly, one step at a time. When the hour-long visit was over, Mrs. Sutton reluctantly placed Tommy back into the incubator and then lingered a few moments. At last, a bond was forming between mother and son.

During the next 4 weeks, we taught Mrs. Sutton suctioning and tracheostomy care by practicing on a doll. When we felt confident of her skills, we insisted she care for Tommy. At first, she was frightened, especially if he cried. (And because of the tracheostomy, Tommy cried soundlessly.) "Am I hurting him?" she'd ask anxiously. We'd assure her she wasn't. Eventually, she began anticipating Tommy's needs even before we did, and she'd remind us when he needed suctioning. Every time she learned a new skill, she'd say, "That wasn't as hard as I thought."

After Mrs. Sutton had mastered all the techniques, we helped her teach Mr. Sutton. Being the teacher not only gave her a chance to practice, but it also helped bring the couple closer together.

The physical therapist taught the Suttons how to do chest physical therapy; and the occupational therapist taught them how to exercise Tommy to strengthen his neck muscles, which had become weak because the tracheostomy tube limited his movement. We also gave the Suttons tips on emergency care and pointers on how to travel safely and comfortably with Tommy. We urged them to teach one of their relatives to care for Tommy, so they'd have more freedom. Then we arranged for a visiting nurse to help out during Tommy's first few weeks at home and gave them a list of all the equipment they'd need and where to buy or rent it.

Two days before Tommy's discharge, we arranged for Mrs. Sutton to spend 24 hours in the hospital. We moved a bed into an empty storage room next to the nursery, to create as independent an environment as possible. Then we moved Tommy and all his paraphernalia into the room. We told Mrs. Sutton we wouldn't disturb her—we wanted her and Tommy to have complete pravacy. Of course, if she had any problems, she knew we were only a buzzer away. She never called us once, although, later on, she admitted she hadn't slept a wink all night.

The Suttons took Tommy home 2 days later. Just before they left the nursery, Mrs. Sutton touched my arm and said shyly, "I can't tell you how much Tommy's letter meant to me. You know we framed it and have it in our living room. Thank you for all your help."

After the Suttons had gone, I couldn't help but think that although we'd used all our sophisticated nursing skills to make Tommy well, what he needed most was his mother's love. But you can't write "love" on your care plan; it has to come from the heart.

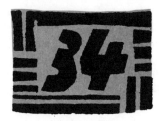

Sam, the Patient Nobody Wanted to Visit

SHARON WARLICK, RN

I'd been out of school for only 6 months and had never cared for a severely burned patient—nor had many of the nurses at our small, community hospital. So when we got our first glimpse of Sam, who was rushed in by helicopter, we were frankly horrified.

Sam, whose occupation was that of prison guard, had been clearing land behind his home. Unthinkingly, he'd thrown gasoline on a stump fire, and the explosion had covered half his body with second- and third-degree burns. His polyester clothes had melted and stuck to his seared flesh. Skin hung in black shreds from his swollen, blistered ears; his hair was gone. In honesty, his head looked like a great lump of charcoal.

Horrified or not, you do your job. And immediately—almost automatically—we started I.V.s and inserted a subclavian line. As soon as Sam's condition stabilized, we moved him upstairs into reverse isolation.

Sam's wife, who was seriously hypertensive, was ordered by her doctor to stay at home. But Sam's daughter and his brother soon arrived in a second helicopter. They were gowned and taken straight to his room. Even though Sam was sedated, he couldn't have missed their reaction. Shocked and revolted by his appearance, they could barely make themselves look at him.

They were the last visitors Sam had for a number of days. Friends and relatives telephoned regularly and many dropped by the hospital. When we offered them a chance to visit Sam in person, however, they became pressed for time, developed colds, or explained that they didn't want to disturb him. Sam got more get-well cards and fewer visitors than anybody else on the floor. Everybody cared about him, but nobody wanted to visit him.

We could hardly blame them. We were almost as horrified by his appearance as they were. It's one thing to sit in a classroom and understand that a patient mustn't think you can't take him as he is. But it's another thing to find tendrils of charred, foul-smelling skin stripping away as you remove a dressing. We'd try hard not to grimace, but we weren't always successful.

Sam's doctor had ordered silver nitrate as the method of treatment. Nothing could have been more difficult and time-consuming, we thought.

First, we had to wrap Sam from the waist up in the soaked dressings. Then we had to cover those with dry ones. Fours hours later, we'd take them all off and wrap him up again. We did that six times a day.

Along with that, he had to be taken to the Hubbard tank for debridement every morning. It wasn't easy finding a way to cover all of Sam's treatments without throwing our regular nursing routine completely out of whack. Still, in a couple of days, we worked out a schedule that fit everything in. We were pretty pleased with ourselves.

The fifth night after he was admitted, Sam's light went on around midnight. Until then he'd been too weak to ask for anything, and the nurse was pleased with this apparent show of progress. Sam asked for a drink of water. The nurse filled a glass, handed it to him, and started to leave. Then, as she heard the glass shatter, she turned to see Sam jump out of bed, brandishing the jagged bottom of the glass. Thinking he meant it for her, she screamed. But, before anyone else could react, Sam slashed both his wrists.

We forgot all about isolation precautions as we rushed into his room. Quickly, we applied pressure to the wrist wounds and the site of the subclavian line he'd pulled out in his frenzy. Sam, exhausted by then, offered no resistance. As we caught our breath and waited for the doctor on call to arrive with suture materials, we were all thinking the same thing. What had we been doing wrong? We should never have been taken so totally unprepared by a patient's behavior.

The next morning, Sam's doctor asked him to talk about what had happened. At first, he simply couldn't. This rugged, self-reliant officer didn't know how to tell anyone how lonely, scared, and depressed he was. However, when an attendant, unaware of what was going on, rolled in a wheelchair for Sam's regular morning debridement session, our patient found the strength to protest.

"No," Sam shouted, "I won't go in there again. They're skinning me alive."

Then the rest of it came out: What was the point of living if no one could stand to look at him? Even his family didn't want to see him. It was like being condemned to solitary confinement—for life. Our treatments only compounded his agony. Why didn't we just let him die?

Later at staff conference, we all discussed what had gone wrong. While we'd been congratulating ourselves on how well we'd met Sam's physical needs, we'd obviously been neglecting his emotional needs. We'd let him be cut off from everything he knew and everyone who could support him.

No, we hadn't initiated his family's feelings of revulsion, but we hadn't done enough to help them overcome them. Our failure had given silent support to their avoidance of Sam and confirmed *his* worst fears about his injury. We spent a while telling ourselves how over-worked and understaffed we were and how we weren't used to cases like Sam's. And certainly, all that was true enough. But it only explained our failure. It didn't excuse it. Clearly, we had to make some changes.

While maintaining the reverse isolation Sam needed for his burns to heal, we had to find a way

"No," Sam shouted before his morning debridement session, "I won't go in there again. They're skinning me alive." Then the rest of it came out: What was the point of living if no one could stand to look at him? Even his family didn't want to see him. It was like being condemned to solitary confinement—for life.

to help him maintain contact with the outside world. First, in order to help him keep track of time, we brought him a clock and a calendar. We had the newspapers autoclaved and brought to his room every day. Every one of us made a special point of helping Sam's family and friends understand how much their visits would mean to him. As each one agreed to try it, we briefed them on exactly what they could expect to see.

When Sam's wife was finally allowed to visit, we helped her overcome her fear by explaining every phase of his treatment and emphasizing every bit of progress he made.

I think a lot of the fright of seeing someone in Sam's condition comes from an unconscious reasoning that anything so awful must be permanent. As soon as we can see some progress, though, we begin to accept the condition as temporary, and it becomes something we can handle. Certainly this is what happened in Sam's case. Every healed blister and every patch of healthy new skin were pointed out to visitors as positive steps in Sam's recovery. As people saw him progress, their feelings of revulsion diminished, and their visits became more frequent.

Sam's doctor helped him master his fear of the debridement sessions by scheduling them every other day so he could rest in between. Furthermore, Sam was told that he was free to call off any session he thought he couldn't face. That was all the challenge he needed. He never missed one after that.

Two days after Sam slashed his wrists, we brought a mirror to his room. Until then, he'd only seen his facial burns reflected in the horrified faces of his family and the grim masks of nurses trying to hide their feelings. Bad as he looked, it was nothing compared to what he'd imagined. When

he saw his own face for the first time, he began to laugh. We thought it might be hysteria until we realized he was laughing out of sheer relief.

"Well sir, I'm not very pretty," he said, "but then, I never was."

From then on, Sam's courage never failed him, and the laughter we heard for the first time that day soon became part of our daily lives.

I especially remember the day I finally got his dressings right. If you've ever wrapped silver nitrate dressings, you know what a mess they are. Forget keeping your uniform and shoes spotless; just try to get home without looking like a dalmatian. We all had to struggle and fumble with Sam's dressings before we got the hang of it. For a while there, I thought I'd never get it right. Finally, the day came when I got him wrapped up perfectly.

"Now we're cooking with gas," I announced proudly. Then I gulped and stammered and blushed. *How could I have said such a thing?*

Well, Sam just roared with laughter. I was so relieved, I joined right in.

That's the kind of man Sam was. That fellow who jumped out of bed with a jagged glass in his hand wasn't the real Sam. That was an aberration caused by pain and despair.

Fortunately, by reestablishing Sam's contact with the world he'd known, by helping his family overcome their fear enough to give him the support he needed, and by letting him use his own courage, we were able to dispel that aberration. We were able to send home a Sam very much like the Sam everyone had known before the accident.

Sarah Wanted to Die at Home, but Her Family Resisted

VICTORIA CHURA, RN

Working with a terminally ill patient presents special problems. Sometimes, it won't be the patient—but the family—who will need the greatest care. I was glad to be on duty during Sarah's last days.

As a visiting nurse in a predominantly rural area, I work with many self-reliant farm people. Unaccustomed to hospitals and frightened by their procedures, they prefer to be cared for at home—no matter what!

One such patient was Sarah, a terminal-cancer patient who insisted on returning home. She had been discharged from the hospital with a Foley catheter. I was sent to instruct the family in catheter care.

Two agitated women greeted me at the door. Their first statement was, "Thank God you're here, she pulled out that tube!" As they hurried me past the living room, they introduced themselves as the patient's daughters-in-law. Nancy, her husband and their five children lived with Sarah. Anne lived close by. Once we were seated in the kitchen they continued. "She is terrible. She just won't listen! They had to tie her in bed when she was in the hospital. How do they expect us to take care of

her? Why did they send her home like this? She was in no condition to come home. We don't know how to take care of someone this bad!"

I asked for more history on the patient and was told that she didn't know she had cancer. A large open lesion had been treated with X-ray therapy, but brain and spine metastasis had been discovered. They showed me the list of low-sodium menus the patient was supposed to follow to prevent cerebal edema. "But," Nancy exclaimed, "she won't eat this stuff!"

When the family seemed more composed, I asked to see the patient. A large double bed had been moved into the living room but as I entered, I saw a strong-looking, 80-year-old woman sitting very straight on a chair. She had raised nine children, had been widowed many years, and was very accustomed to having things done her way. Staying in bed was not her way.

The daughter-in-law announced, "Here's the nurse, mom. She'll make you listen!" I could have wished for a less challenging introduction as the patient looked at me long and hard—taking my measure. After a few moments of silence, I smiled, introduced myself and said, "The hospital said you wanted to go home. They asked me to stop by and help out a bit." She extended her hand to me, stating, "My name is Sarah." As she held my hand, she gently pulled me toward her, indicating that I sit beside her.

"When you come, I want you to come in here, okay, nurse? I can't hear what you say when you're out there. I didn't mean to pull that tube out. I was sleeping, I felt something down there, before I knowed what I was doing, I pulled it out. I didn't mean it, nurse, honest!"

I smiled and said, "Sometimes things like that happen. We can put in another one. But, you'll have to try to remember it's there and not pull it out anymore." Still holding my hand she promised, "Oh, I won't, nurse!"

I wanted to know for myself how much Sarah knew of her condition. I asked her to tell me why she had gone to the hospital. "I had this big sore," she said indicating the area of the lesion. "They gave me treatments, and it went away from here. But, I can feel it inside me. They did all they could for me, nurse." She didn't use the word *cancer* but I felt that this shrewd, old farm woman had sized up the situation.

"They was feeding me through my veins, but I knowed they wasn't going to make me better, so I pulled the tubes out. I wanted to go home and they tied me in my bed. I told them I could take my pain pills at home, then they let me go home."

"Yeah," said the daughter-in-law, "but you won't eat!"

"I can't eat that stuff, it don't taste no good!" the patient said.

I thought we ought to get the question of diet settled right away, so I called their family doctor. His advice was: "Give her what she will eat, just don't add any salt to her foods." That settled, I proceeded with the catheter instructions.

The next morning, I received a call from Nancy. The catheter was not draining, they were unable to irrigate it, and the patient was complaining of pain in her lower abdomen. There was a small amount of milky white urine in the drainage bag. "All she would drink was buttermilk—over a gallon of buttermilk."

I told her that I would be right out to change the catheter, and I asked her to purchase a supply of cranberry juice.

Families find it very hard to deny the dying patient anything. When the patient's wishes start causing more discomfort or pain, however, the family must take a firm stand. The backing of professional opinion will give them strong support.

When I got there, I said, "Sarah, you can't just drink buttermilk, you have to drink and eat other things, too. Calcium in the buttermilk is clogging up your catheter. I want you to start drinking cranberry juice." I then explained to the family that the cranberry juice would produce a more acid urine, with less chance for sediment and infection. I suggested that they use the buttermilk as a reward only after the patient had eaten a reasonable amount of other food. The following day the urine was much clearer.

A few days later, the family called to say that Sarah had taken a convulsion in the night and was admitted to the hospital unconscious. Two days later, I received another call. "Can you come back? The hospital called us last night at 11:00, to come and get her. She refused to stay and they weren't going to keep her there against her will."

When I knocked, I was led out to the kitchen where a number of Sarah's children were having a heated discussion. "Why did they send her home? She is in no condition to come home. We want our mother to have the best of care. Call the ambulance and send her back!" Everyone in the family got a chance to air his opinion—except Sarah. I thought this called for a patient-advocate.

When there was a break in the conversation, I asked, "Have you talked to your mother? Did you ask her what *she* wants? Go in and talk to her. Tell her you would feel better if she were in the hospital. If you can convince her to go, then I'll call the ambulance. But no ambulance is going to take out some poor old lady who's kicking and screaming, 'I don't want to go!' And no hospital is going to keep her against her will."

A period of silence followed. No one was eager to approach Sarah. She was still a formidable figure.

Finally, one son went into the room to talk and we heard Sarah say, "No, I want to stay here! They did all they can for me. I can stay here and die if I want to."

This is a hard decision for any family to accept. Humanly enough, they would like to be relieved of the enormous burden of caring for a dying person. And, honestly enough, they believe that the hospital will provide better care.

Families need a great deal of support at this time. They turned to me for direction. "What do you say, nurse?" I told them I thought they would make the right decision in fulfilling their mother's last wishes. Sarah would die more peacefully at home, and she would get the best of care. Our Home Nursing Service would make daily visits. We would instruct and supervise the family in all aspects of Sarah's care. When the family dispersed, they were somber, but also, I think, relieved.

As the days passed, Sarah became increasingly confused. Nancy wanted to have her annointed, but was afraid this gesture would alert Sarah to the fact that she was dying. I felt Sarah already knew this, so I told Nancy that perhaps Sarah thought she was protecting *them* from the knowledge of her approaching death.

In one of her more lucid moments, I asked, "Sarah, is it all right if we call the priest? Your family would feel better if you were to receive the Sacrament of the Sick. And, you may feel better, too." The patient looked at her family shrewdly and consented. I think it was then she realized that the others knew she was dying. For a few days after the priest's visit, Sarah was reported to be "as good as gold."

A few days later, however, as I approached the house, I heard a great commotion in the patient's room. I hurried in to find the family desperately trying to hold Sarah in bed. She kept repeating, "I have to get up, I have to get up!" I came over, took her hand, and said, "Sarah, why do you have to get up?"

"I have to take care of Tommy," she answered. "Who's Tommy?" I asked Nancy. "Her youngest son," she answered reluctantly. "He's mentally retarded. He's been her chief concern for over 30 years." "Where is he?" I asked. "Upstairs."

I told the family that the dying—despite all logic—feel guiltily responsible for leaving tasks undone. I thought Sarah's concern for Tommy's future explained her present turmoil.

A few moments lapsed, then Nancy said, "Sarah was always afraid we'd put him in the County Home if she died. But my husband and I were talking about it last night. We're going to keep him at home with us."

"Did you tell her that?" I asked. "But she's too confused," Nancy protested. "You'd be surprised at how much can get through," I said. "Try."

Nancy hesitated, then took Sarah's hand. "Mom, don't worry about Tommy. We'll take care of him. We won't put Tommy in the County Home." Almost immediately Sarah ceased struggling, and lay back relaxed. I motioned for Nancy to come out into the kitchen.

I encouraged her to talk to Tommy, to help prepare him for the eventuality of his mother's death. Too often in our preoccupation with the dying, we neglect the needs of the living. Tommy, especially with his handicap, should be prepared.

The next day, I met Tommy for the first time. He was sitting on a chair next to Sarah's bed. She looked up and smiled proudly. "This is my boy, Tommy, nurse." Tommy just looked at me as I said, "Hi." He broke a piece from the sandwich he was eating, gave it to his mother, and Sarah, who had been refusing all food, munched on it contentedly.

Toward the end of the fourth week, Nancy phoned excitedly. "White stuff is coming from her

 They were silent as I spoke, yet I seemed to feel it was something they all needed to hear. "Many times," I said, "patients are ready to die, yet they hold on until they can sense things have been settled and they can leave in peace— that you won't go all to pieces."

mouth. I called the doctor and he's coming, but I forgot to ask him what to do until he gets here."

I told her to position Sarah on her side, as I had shown her previously, and to wipe the mucus as it drained from her mouth.

When I got there, the doctor had just left. "She's dying. The doctor said she's dying; it's just a matter of time," Nancy stated as I entered the kitchen. "It's just Anne and me here. I've never seen anyone die before. My husband went to work this morning. I'm so mad! It's his mother! He said he didn't want to see her die." Nancy was bordering on hysteria and it was going to be a long day. I sat her down, made a cup of tea and let her talk out her fears and frustration. When she'd finished, I said, "Maybe it's better he did go to work. Some people can't endure seeing their mother die. Besides, you and Anne have been with Sarah the most. She feels most secure with the two of you."

I went to check Sarah's vital signs. There was no discernible blood pressure, the pulse was weak, rapid and thready, her breathing labored. Standing beside me at the bedside, Anne said, "They say that hearing is the last thing to leave us, perhaps she can still hear. Maybe we should go into the kitchen to talk."

"But, Sarah always liked to hear what was being said," I reminded her. Standing there watching each labored breath couldn't help, however. I suggested they go get a cup of coffee, and sit and talk in the room. Sarah would sense their presence and be comforted. We were quiet for awhile, then Anne asked how long I thought it would be. I placed my hand on Sarah's. "I think she is ready to go now.

Perhaps what she needs to know is that it will be alright with you."

They were silent as I spoke, yet I seemed to feel it was something they all needed to hear. "Many times," I said, "patients are ready to die, yet they hold on until they can sense things have been settled and they can leave in peace—that you won't go all to pieces."

I directed our talk into a calm discussion of what they might do when Sarah died. I told them that some families want the doctor to come and make an official pronouncement of death. Others want a priest. I explained how to remove the catheter and prepare the body before the undertaker arrived. Most of all, I encouraged them to support their husbands. At a time like this, even the seemingly strongest of men need support. In a while, Sarah's respirations quieted considerably; she seemed in peace and unafraid. I asked the family to call me if they needed me, that I would be returning to the office.

When I got there, I found a telephone message. Sarah had died 5 minutes after I'd left.

As I added this to the case report, I thought of how hard it is to conceive that the dying need permission to do the inevitable. Yet there it was, spread out before me in the case records.

It wasn't until Sarah knew the family knew she was dying; knew her unfinished task (Tommy) would be taken care of; and knew the family could accept her leaving, that she could let go in peace.

The Gordons Needed all the Help They Could Get

MARIE SCOTT BROWN, RN, PhD

Most nurses' work philosophy could roughly be summed up as: *Patient plus nurse equals healing, and healing equals success*. But what if no healing is possible... if the patient's condition is irreversible? What then becomes our goal? By what standards do we measure success? These were questions I had to face in my work with the Gordons.

I was a pediatric nurse practitioner in a Denver city clinic when I first met the Gordons. Jack Gordon, an education major, was in his senior year at the local university. Jane, his wife, was an attractive, bubbly 21-year-old. She was also intelligent, and I wondered why she had waited until she was well into her sixth month of pregnancy before seeking prenatal care. She would have come sooner, she explained, but she'd been out of the state for 4 months, caring for her dying mother.

Still, Jane was young and healthy, and the detailed history I took suggested no problems ahead. The labor was easy and the delivery, normal. But Jamey, their sturdy, 8-pound son, was born with such minimal sight and hearing that he is technically blind and deaf.

After the birth of a defective child, parents go through a grieving process—denial, anger, depression—not unlike that of families who are preparing for a member's death. I saw the Gordons going through these stages and, despite their sessions with our clinic psychiatrist, I knew they would have to work through to acceptance themselves.

When Jamey was 6 months old, we had him fitted with a hearing aid and powerful glasses so he could make the best use of the slight vision and hearing he had. Little by little, I saw both parents starting to get satisfaction from being able to parent Jamey successfully. I felt they were reaching a stage of acceptance.

When Jamey was 1 year old, Jack graduated and got a teaching job in rural Arkansas. The last time I saw the Gordons, we talked honestly. They knew they had a big job ahead of them, but they felt—as did I—that some way they'd be able to handle it.

Two years later, I walked into the clinic to find a tired, worn-looking woman sitting listlessly in a chair. A little boy in diapers crawled around on the floor alternately making high-pitched screeching noises and sucking pureed food out of a bottle with a large hole in the nipple. Every so often, he would stop crawling and sit, rocking back and forth while rhythmically poking at his eyes. Almost a full minute passed before I recognized Jane and Jamey Gordon.

During that first visit, the most I could do was listen. Although Jane spoke in an emotionless monotone, her story described the devastation of three lives.

The Gordons had returned to Denver so Jack could get his master's degree. They expected this to take about 2 years, but Jane didn't expect the change in scene to solve the desperate situation they were in. They were, quite simply, overwhelmed by Jamey's needs.

At 3 years of age, he still couldn't walk; the only solid food he would take was pureed food sucked from the nipple of a bottle; he wasn't toilet-trained; he slept only 4 to 5 hours out of every 24, and these were unpredictably spaced out over night and day. He refused to wear his hearing aid or glasses, pulling them off the minute he felt them on his head; he demonstrated no affection and frequently hit out, bit, and screamed when approached; he spent most of his waking hours head-banging, thumb-sucking, and masturbating.

Living in a remote section of the country, the Gordons had few resources to turn to for help. The one time they'd had Jamey evaluated for possible mental retardation, the doctors were unable to determine whether his behavior was caused by retardation or by lack of sensory input.

Jane was silent after this long recitation. Then suddenly she screamed, "I hate him, I hate him." Appalled by what she'd said, she burst into tears.

Whe she regained control, I started to probe gently about the rest of her life—her time away from Jamey. Then, it was my turn to be appalled. *Jane had no time away from Jamey.*

Since no babysitter could care for Jamey, the Gordons had him 24 hours a day. Even his crib was in their bedroom because they feared for his safety. More important, Jack had begun to work longer and longer hours overtime. Jane (correctly, I thought) interpreted this as his way of escaping the problem. She was openly angry at having Jack "dump" Jamey on her.

At the end of the session, I suggested we next meet at the Gordons' home so I could see Jamey

in his usual surroundings. I selected a date 2 weeks from that day because, as I confessed to Jane, I felt I needed all the time I could get to try to find some handle on the Gordons' problems. Jane's last words were that she felt better for just having talked to me. I, quite honestly, felt overwhelmed.

That evening, after much telephoning to colleagues who had experience with handicapped children, I decided the most direct course of action would be to contact the university's department of special education. The next day, I learned that not only did the department have students specializing in the education of deaf-blind children, but it also sponsored a program of field work for senior students. If the Gordons were interested, a student would work directly with Jamey. The school also held a daily, 2-hour class for deaf-blind children; the only requirement was that the child be toilet-trained. Further, for the parents of handicapped children, the school sponsored a weekly discussion group led by an experienced social worker. I felt I'd come across a gold mine.

When I called Jane with my news, she welcomed having a student's help. So, on the appointed day, Allie, the student, joined Jane and me at the Gordons' home.

I had asked Jane to write down all her problems in the order of their priority. Admittedly, her list was formidable—but it concerned only Jamey. As a nurse, I felt Jane had overlooked her most basic problem: her own energy level. Until Jane could get proper rest, she wouldn't have the energy to keep up with Jamey.

Allie and I worked out a plan to "cycle" Jamey into a more normal schedule by helping him differentiate between day and night. Jamey, like most deaf-blind children, could distinguish some light and sound. During the day, Jane was to keep Jamey in the brightest room in the house. She also was to turn on all the lights in the room and play the radio loudly from time to time. At night, she would keep Jamey as calm and quiet as possible. For this, she would have to move him into the second bedroom, which would be made as dark and sound-proof as possible. We also suggested that she have him sleep in his playpen. Since Jamey slept so little, he'd need the extra room of a playpen to move around in when he awoke.

At the end of a week, Allie and I met with the

Gordons. They both agreed that the new arrangement gave them somewhat more rest, but Jack was still reluctant to give Jane the other hours she needed for herself. He insisted that he had to work in the library almost every night. We finally convinced him that he could at least mind Jamey for 2 hours a week so Jane could attend the meetings for parents of handicapped children.

Those meetings were probably the best thing that had happened to Jane since Jamey's birth. From them, she learned that Jamey's behavior was typical of the deaf-blind child. All the other parents had suffered through their children's delayed walking and toilet training—the rhythmic poking at the eyes, thumb-sucking, and masturbation. Now, all those children were in class. None was judged retarded.

Parents whose children had made the class paired off with parents whose children hadn't yet reached that level. Mrs. Chavez, whose deaf-blind child had progressed somewhat beyond Jamey, came to the Gordons. And a wonderful thing happened: Jane relearned how to play with her son—something she hadn't done since he was a small baby.

The deaf-blind child has a strong tactile sense, and Mrs. Chavez brought Play-doh, clay, and simple objects such as spoons, building blocks, swatches of material, and sponges to provide the contrast of big to small, smooth to rough, and wet to dry. With Mrs. Chavez' encouragement and with Jane holding him for safety, Jamey got to know and like the sensation of the sliding board, teeter-totter, and swing.

Soon, Jane began to invent games for Jamey. She made a huge, 4-piece, plywood puzzle and spent hours teaching him how to work it. Once he learned, he'd spend as long as a half hour quietly working it together and apart.

Then she altered her household chores to give Jamey different experiences. For example, she postponed doing the daily dishes until after the last meal. Then, as she washed the day's pile, Jamey played in the sink beside her, enjoying the water games with varied-shaped sponges and floating and sinking balls. She began to vacuum daily because Jamey loved to hold onto the vacuum

cleaner, ear pressed tightly against it, enjoying the vibrations and the motor's roar.

Jamey's acceptance of anything new came very slowly and all these experiences took many months. We were surprised, then, when his ability to walk came almost miraculously. When I left him one week, he was still crawling; the next, he was walking almost as well as a sighted child.

Our next biggest hurdle was toilet training. I had Jane keep a record of Jamey's bowel movements for a month. We could trace a definite pattern, and Jane would put him on a potty chair at the appropriate times. Every time he had a bowel movement on the potty, she rewarded him with two spoonfuls of ice cream. Once he learned to take food from a spoon (and that took some doing, too), the spoonfuls of ice cream became an important part of reinforcing desirable behavior. Jamey really loved ice cream.

Once Jamey was admitted into the class, he progressed at an acceptable pace. Then the time came for another decision. Jack got his master's degree. The Gordons had to weigh Jamey's need for special education against Jack's career opportunities. They compromised by returning to Arkansas for the school year and by spending the summers in Denver, where the three of them attend a program for handicapped children and their parents.

The Gordons stopped in to see me when they returned for their first summer's program. I was pleased to see that Jamey was learning sign language. I was even more pleased to see Jamey sidle up to his mother and comfortably finger her hand or sleeve. Jane, in turn, did more cuddling and hugging than I'd ever seen her do before. I guess my biggest thrill was to see Jamey's smile. His daddy leaned over and chucked him on the cheek, and for the first time, I saw Jamey smile.

Jamey was the first deaf-blind child I had ever worked with but, when I think of the Gordons, I have a real sense of accomplishment. We had managed to set realistic goals for both the levels of Jamey's performance and the time it would take to reach them.

That little boy's smile is my idea of success.

The Man Who Knew too Much

DIANA WILKIEMEYER, RN, MS

In patient teaching, one of our first problems is trying to scale down the information to the layman's level. But what if the person we're teaching "knows too much"? That calls for an about-face in our approach. And that's not always easy to do, as we learned in our dealings with Mr. Mellon.

Mr. Mellon, let me explain, was not the patient—his wife was. Mrs. Mellon, 60 years old, had fallen while traveling in Central America with her sister. Later, when she became comatose and was hospitalized, her condition was misdiagnosed as "insulin coma." Eventually, she was flown back to the United States where the doctors diagnosed her condition as cerebral hemorrhage and performed a craniotomy to relieve pressure on the brain. The surgery saved her life but also left her a right-side hemiplegic. She was disoriented with grossly impaired speech.

Mrs. Mellon spent 1 month in a hospital and a total of 6 hours in a nursing home before her husband, raging against the "total incompetence" of all health-care workers (from neurosurgeons to aides), took her back to their apartment.

At this point, I, as a visiting nurse, began my work with the Mellons. Mrs. Mellon's condition was something of a puzzle. She couldn't perceive pain or vibration in her right leg; her right arm was spastic and in flexion—except for the fingers. Her speech was garbled and she didn't respond to her name or to any vocal command. Yet often, when familiar items (spoon, comb, toothbrush) were placed in front of her, she could use them properly—albeit awkwardly. Sometimes she was agitated, and bit and fought people. Other times, she was pleasantly cooperative. Her condition was indeed complicated.

Mr. Mellon's condition was also complicated. He desperately wanted help for his wife, but his manner was so hostile and intellectually intimidating that he turned off all would-be helpers.

He was a retired electrical engineer and he had what amounted to a mania for finding out *why* things work as they do. Before we could even get to see the patient, we first were put through a session that seemed like an oral exam.

Mr. Mellon would sit and study his wife for hours, jotting down notes on any pattern in her jumbled speech, any reaction to stimuli—television, recordings, family photographs. Then when we nurses appeared, we'd be barraged with rapid-fire questions.

Why would his wife show animation at a profile picture of her cousin and not at a full-face picture of the same woman? *Was* there still a swelling in his wife's brain; *would* it gradually subside? *Were* new nerve pathways being set up in her brain? *Would* she ever regain bladder function... be able to stand alone... talk to him sensibly?

He could barely contain his scorn when we had to answer most of his questions with an honest "nobody really knows."

His technical questions were even more difficult to handle. What was the anatomic structure of the axon cells—their synaptic junction? What's the latest research on acetylcholine and dopamine in impulse transmission?

Then, maddeningly enough, when we would go to a lot of trouble calling sources or doing library research, to try to answer one of his questions, he *always* challenged the answer. *Always.* "That's not what Miss X says," he'd maintain, naming one of our co-workers. Or he'd quote from a text that gave a variation—or refutation—of the answer we'd just gone to so much trouble to find.

Mr. Mellon antagonized everyone who worked with him—from the home aide, to the speech therapist, to the physiatrist. But recognizing that still didn't help *our* morale.

At a nursing conference, we all took turns describing the frustrating experiences we'd had with Mr. Mellon. Frankly, we saw him as an annoying hurdle in our path to the patient, but we knew that he was a *permanent* hurdle. In order to work with Mrs. Mellon, we had to work through him. So, if only for our patient's sake, we had to remember the man's good qualities. And they *were* good qualities—high intelligence, keen observation, unquestioned devotion.

We decided that our best approach was to make a complete about-face and try to think of ourselves as fortunate to have such an intelligent, observant colleague who was on 24-hour duty with our patient. *Colleague*—that would be our new approach. We'd let him know how much we relied on him, and how much we valued his opinions and observations. We'd try to follow through on *his* suggestions and always use proper medical terminol-

ogy. We would also assign only one nurse to the case. That way, Mr. Mellon wouldn't feel put upon because he repeatedly had to explain his thought to a succession of people. Further, one nurse would be more likely to notice the small changes that indicate progress in a hemiplegic patient. I was to be that nurse.

Privately, I added one more condition. I promised myself I wouldn't take Mr. Mellon's comments personally. Not his acerbic comments on all health-care workers or his despairing cry of "Nobody helps. I have to do it all alone. You can't rely on anybody."

The new plan had good effects almost immediately. For example, once when I was changing the patient's plugged catheter, Mr. Mellon wanted to know why it plugged so often. I gave him the used one, just as I would to a colleague, so he could study its function. He noted where the crystals lodged. Within a few days, he found that if he manipulated the tube to crush the crystals, then immediately irrigated the tube, it could go several weeks without being changed.

Encouraged by this small success, he determined that his wife would regain bladder control. None of the professionals I consulted were very encouraging—after all, Mrs. Mellon couldn't even communicate. Still, I did the library work, checking out recommended bladder control techniques—like clamping the catheter for a few hours to build up bladder capacity, or removing the catheter for a few days at a time.

But Mr. Mellon didn't approve. He wanted the catheter out permanently. His wife had been super fastidious all of her life, he explained. He planned to rely on that deeply ingrained trait—and a detailed chart of his own making, tracing her pattern of incontinence.

Once again I deferred to him the same way I would if I were dealing with a respected colleague. I taught him to use clean rags and newspapers to make heavy pads that were much more absorbent than commercial disposable diapers. Mr. Mellon changed the pads as soon as they became the slightest bit damp, and he kept meticulous records. Still, weeks went by without much success.

I suggested a bedside commode, but once again, he had his own way of doing things. He believed that if he provided the familiar setting of the family bathroom, his wife's reeducation would come more easily. So four times a day, at precisely the same time, he'd struggle to transfer his wife into a wheelchair, from the wheelchair to the toilet, then back into the wheelchair. Mr. Mellon was a small man, well into his 60s, and it was exhausting work. But he seemed indefatigable.

And finally, he was rewarded. One day, he brought out his records to show me. Mrs. Mellon had had 5 successive days of continence—she was well on her way to bladder control. "Now, the leg," he said to me intensely. "My wife will walk again." With a man like Mr. Mellon, you just *had* to believe.

But hard? The going was *hard*. Mr. Mellon had set the goal: Once every waking hour, Mrs. Mellon would walk the length of her room. What this amounted to, really, was dragging/carrying her. And not only could she not cooperate in shifting weight, but she usually fought the whole procedure. Then, during this hectic scene, we still had to keep checking for signs—"Was that muscle action from the left hip, or was it propulsion from the motion of the other leg? Please check," Mr. Mellon would shout.

This went on for many months, and finally the hard work and intensity of dedication took its toll. I arrived at the apartment one day to find Mr. Mellon sitting in an armchair, a small, beaten man. "Even *my* nervous energy has its limits," he said sadly. "I don't know. I just don't know."

I suggested he take the afternoon off—go to a movie, or visit someone. The aide and I would handle Mrs. Mellon's walking session. But his nature wouldn't let him disrupt a schedule, so we struggled through our usual session.

After the exertion of walking Mrs. Mellon back and forth, we stopped to catch our breath. We placed Mrs. Mellon's normal hand on the bed's side rail so she would stand on her own for a moment. Suddenly, still chattering incomprehensibly, she walked the length of the bed by herself. Unmistakably, she wanted the wheelchair. We couldn't believe it—she was walking *and* communicating! For the first time in all those desperate months, I saw Mr. Mellon cry. He embraced his wife, whispered, "There is a future, there is."

In the following months, Mrs. Mellon learned to walk with only standby help, and she could climb a short flight of stairs with assistance. Her speech was still garbled and her arm was still spastic, but no one was complaining. She had come such a long way.

The Mellons' case is closed, as far as my work is concerned. But the lesson I learned from it will always be a part of my life.

Nursing is working with people and, as such, will always present us with many unknowns—people's deep needs, hidden strengths. Only when we came to terms with this truth were we able to see Mr. Mellon as a helper—not a hurdle—and one of the most dedicated colleagues a nurse could have.

The Family Loved Sammy but Hated Each Other

LORI CARLEY, RN

There's a saying that 90% of pediatric care is parents—giving them support, answering their questions, helping them cope. An exaggeration, to be sure. But not all that much in the case of Sammy and his family. Their relationships were so bizarre it was as if a soap opera had walked off the screen and onto our unit.

Sammy was a 4-year-old who suffered from a brain stem glioma. He'd been comatose for 2 days when he was brought onto our oncology unit for terminal care. His father and maternal grandmother took turns sitting quietly with him, holding his hand. The few times his father, Mr. Quester, spoke to us, he seemed hostile. But we chalked this up to grief.

We got our first inkling of some of the problems we'd encounter when the charge nurse told us what the oncologist, Dr. DuBois, had learned about Sammy's family. His mother had left before he was diagnosed; the couple divorced, and the mother had remarried. The children—Sammy had three brothers—were living with Mr. Quester.

"Sammy's father believes that Sammy 'caught cancer' because his mother wasn't around," the charge nurse said. "He won't listen to reason. The grandmother is torn between being angry at the father for not taking good care of Sammy and at her daughter for having left him. The fact is, they all seem to hate each other but love that boy."

The frightening part, she added, was that the grandmother had warned her that Mr. Quester could become violent when provoked. "So be careful, okay?"

That we were. Because the father and grandmother rarely spoke to us, we concentrated solely on Sammy's needs. Treatment included high-protein feedings by nasogastric (NG) tube, dexamethasone (Decadron) to minimize cerebral edema, and turning him frequently to prevent decubiti.

Several days later, Sammy came out of his coma, banging on the bedrail and mumbling, "ice cream." Thrilled, we quickly blended some and managed to get a little into him. He remained conscious, though he didn't speak again.

That night, Sammy's mother, Sally, arrived during visiting hours. Her ex-husband was there at the time.

"Hello," I said. "You've come at a good time—Sammy's better today."

"Well, she *left* at a bad time!" Mr. Quester snarled, and stormed out.

Sally looked so panicky I thought she was going to bolt, too. I took hold of her hand. The mental image I'd had of a woman who had callously abandoned her children was fading. She looked like a forlorn little girl.

Though his parents seemed to hate the sight of each other, Sammy loved to see them both. You could tell by his little grin—a grin I came to treasure. So I worked out a visiting schedule to be sure his parents wouldn't meet. Sally agreed to come only during the day; Mr. Quester, only in the evening.

By the end of 2 weeks we were able to remove Sammy's intravenous line. He seemed dysphasic, unable to complain of pain, so he'd only nod or shake his head when we asked. One afternoon, while Sally and her mother were there, he gave me that slight nod. As I began to pour his pain medication into his NG tube, his grandmother grabbed my hand. "He doesn't need that junk, nurse."

Sally explained that her mother was afraid he'd become addicted. When I suggested that Sally discuss this with Dr. DuBois, she said, "I didn't know he'd talk to me."

I was bewildered. Dr. DuBois had spent hours talking to Mr. Quester, and I'd assumed he'd done the same with Sally. But she had been too timid to approach him. After I brought this up with Dr. DuBois, Sally had as much voice in Sammy's care as her husband did.

Sammy's condition, meanwhile, improved daily. Although his prognosis remained the same, his nutritional problems alone kept him in the hospital. Dr. DuBois told us he would send Sammy home for at least a while if we could get him to take enough nourishment by mouth.

We contacted the hospital social worker, and she arranged for Sammy to stay with his father and for his maternal grandmother to come take care of him. She even set up visiting times for Sally.

Meanwhile, we worked at getting Sammy's NG tube removed. The problem wasn't his appetite; his large doses of Decadron ensured that it was

healthy. But the glioma had impaired his swallowing mechanism.

Sammy could handle ice cream and baby food by taking small bites. But unexpectedly, the family hinted that they couldn't afford the extra expense of the baby food. We had to find substitutes.

Taking our cue from the ice cream, we froze

"Sammy's father believes that Sammy 'caught cancer' because his mother wasn't around," the charge nurse said. "He won't listen to reason. The grandmother is torn between being angry at the father for not taking good care of Sammy and at her daughter for having left him. They hate each other but love that boy."

Sammy's high-protein drink until it was like slush. It went down fine. We then worked meats into his diet by mixing them with mashed potatoes and milk. Pasta, after a whirl in the blender, was no problem either.

We had to keep cheering him on while we fed him: "Swallow, Sammy, swallow. That's a good boy." We kept a simple record of what he could and couldn't swallow so his family would know what to give him at home. For instance, peas with hard shells, no matter how well blended, were out, but blended squash was fine.

Strangely, as Sammy got better, his family stopped coming in. After 2 weeks, the social worker drove to the father's home, then reported back that he'd been evicted and that Sammy's brothers were with Sally and her husband. More-over, the grandmother told the social worker that she didn't think she could handle Sammy's care.

Sammy would have to stay with us. We tried our best to be a substitute family for him. Every day, we would roll his crib out by the nurses' station, or sometimes wheel him around in a little wagon as we made rounds. We began teaching him to feed himself; we worked on helping him learn colors and numbers all over again. Even a nurse from the intensive care unit, who'd come to know Sammy just from passing through the hallway, would spend some of her breaks reading to him. That's the kind of child he was (and the kind of staff we have here).

But we knew being in a good home, even a foster home, would be best for him. When the social worker suggested this to Mr. Quester, how-ever, he refused, and the child protection agency could find no legal reason to place Sammy. He wasn't being abused or neglected; his family sim-ply wasn't ready for him. In fact, one evening, with tears in his eyes, Mr. Quester told me, "I just can't manage yet. Please take good care of my boy until I can."

A few days later, 3 months after Sammy was admitted, Mr. Quester did take him home; a home health nurse would help with his care. He also collected Sammy's brothers from Sally. For a few weeks, we heard through the oncology clinic that Sammy was doing well. But a month later, word came from the social worker that Mr. Quester and the children were missing from their home. Sally had no idea where they were either.

Then, after 2 more weeks, Sally called us. Her ex-husband had literally left Sammy and his broth-ers on her doorstep, saying he'd been evicted again and couldn't take care of them. Sally immediately brought Sammy to the hospital. "I just can't stand to watch him suffer anymore," she told us.

We were shocked by Sammy's condition. He was completely aphasic and had lost nearly all use of his limbs. His body was bloated almost beyond recognition. Although he could still swallow, he now had to be spoon-fed.

Because he was so bloated, skin care was a real problem. He had a yeast infection on his scrotum. He moaned when we changed him, since we had to roll him from side to side. It took two of us to

turn him. But an air-fluidized bed helped greatly. Indeed, as he lay on it, he gave us that little grin.

A few evenings after Sally brought Sammy in, Mr. Quester showed up when Sally, her husband Larry, and her mother were there. Suddenly, we heard loud voices, and ran in the room just in time to see Mr. Quester dash some soda into Larry's face. We called on the intercom for security, but by the time the guards got there, Mr. Quester was throwing punches at Larry.

Security sent for the police; they escorted Mr. Quester to his car. A legal order was obtained forbidding him to come to the hospital. But we urged him to call to talk to Sammy.

Several days later, another episode in this human drama occurred. Sally told me she'd given her three sons back to her ex-husband.

"But *why*?" I asked.

"Larry said he couldn't take care of them if I was up here. H-he's really a good man; he'll take care of my children some day, but it's too much now."

I had a long talk with her, urged her to go to the social worker for help. About a week after that, the social worker told me Sally had started group therapy. The picture that was emerging of her first marriage was a harrowing one: She'd fled from her husband's beatings and had remarried so she could make a home for her children.

One evening, I bumped into Sally in the snack bar. "I know you think I'm terrible," she said, "but I'm torn. I want to visit my son, but I want this marriage to work."

"I don't think you're terrible," I said. "You're someone who has problems. But I also know Sammy enjoys your visits."

"Do you?" she exclaimed. "You don't think he blames me for being sick?"

I stared at her in amazement. Then it hit me that she actually believed what her ex-husband had told her: That, by leaving, she'd as much as "given" Sammy cancer. Terrible feelings of guilt were be-hind her erratic behavior.

"Oh, Sammy," she suddenly wept, "I'm so sorry."

I led her across the hall to the chapel, telling her over and over that she hadn't caused Sammy's illness, trying to assure her that he loved her. "Sally, you have a right to visit your son. And he needs you."

Gradually, she stopped crying. I had to go back to work, but I told her I would ask the chaplain to see her.

She didn't visit Sammy for a couple days—and we were worried. But when she showed up, she was obviously different. She helped with such things as straightening his sheets and changing him—things she'd never done before. She also spoke to him more as a mother than a timid visitor.

Meanwhile, Mr. Quester was calling every day; he'd speak to Sammy while we held the phone to the child's ear. Because these conversations always brightened Sammy's spirits, we encouraged them. Yet I wondered if Sally, so hurt by her ex-husband, would resent Sammy's feelings about him. But I needn't have worried.

I walked into Sammy's room one day to see her helping Sammy with the phone. She was saying, "Daddy wants to tell you 'Hi.' " A few minutes later, she said into the phone: "He's smiling. Thank you for calling."

Sally and Sammy had about a month together. She would sing lullabies to him, sometimes while brushing his hair or rubbing his back or just hold-ing his hand. And she stayed with him most nights. It was as though she were trying to give him a lifetime of mothering.

As happens so often, death came in the early morning hours when only the staff was there. We met Sally at the door to Sammy's room when she returned. Wet-eyed but strong, she asked to use the phone. She apparently called her mother, who soon appeared with Mr. Quester.

Although she spoke quietly to them, there was a firmness in her voice as she talked about such things as whom to call and which funeral director to use. They seemed surprised by this "new woman" and listened attentively to what she said.

A couple weeks later we got the good news that Sally's husband had joined her in therapy—and that Mr. Quester was seeing a therapist, too.

As our charge nurse had told us on the day Sammy was admitted, the one thing this family had in common, despite all their problems, was their love for the boy. And how he loved them. Perhaps that's why, when I think of how we were able to help them—how Sally, in particular, grew as a person through her son's ordeal—I never fail to think of that little grin.

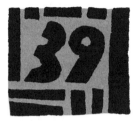

Lottie Tried to Do Everything for Her Husband — Including Our Job

LINDA ROBERTS, RN
ELAINE KENISTON, CNA, BEd

The road to recovery is seldom smooth, and the support of a spouse or close friend can make the journey easier. But *too much* loving attention can actually hamper a patient's recovery.

When a manipulative wife—like Lottie—attempts to take care of all her husband's needs, she robs him of a prime healthy motivation: his desire for independence. Without that, the patient remains little more than a dependent child.

We'll admit it. Picturing Mr. Heller, an 83-year-old diabetic, as a child isn't easy. At 6 feet 1 inch (182.5 cm) and 250 pounds (112.5 kg), with a shock of steel-gray hair on his head, he seemed more like a big old polar bear. Sometimes he was just as tough to manage.

Besides diabetes, Mr. Heller had cerebral atherosclerosis, bilateral neuropathy of both legs, a dry decubitus ulcer on his left heel, severe footdrop in both feet, and partial contracture of his hands. After spending 2 months in the hospital for prostate surgery, he required daily nursing care at home.

For us, that meant driving 10 miles (16 km) from town to his three-room house in the New Hampshire mountains and 10 miles back again,

three times every day. Nonambulatory, Mr. Heller needed our help just to get out of bed. He was so cumbersome that it took two aides to stand-pivot-sit transfer him to his wheelchair. Naturally, his wife Lottie, at 80 years old, couldn't move him by herself. But she sure wanted to do everything else for him.

Like the mountain woman of lore, Lottie insisted on taking total charge. She tried to control every aspect of her husband's home care. With her long, silver hair and squat, rugged body, she reminded us of a chunk of granite, indomitable and utterly self-contained. What she lacked in strength, she made up for in boundless determination.

Besides preparing all his meals, cleaning the house, and doing most of the laundry in an antiquated wringer-type machine, Lottie gave her husband his daily insulin injections. She also emptied his bedpan and urinal and tested his urine. Since all their hot water had to be heated over a wood-burning stove, she had a full day of work ahead of her each morning.

Lottie prided herself on how well she catered to her husband's needs, but her kindness had a cutting edge. For instance, she'd spoon-feed him breakfast in bed every morning although he was capable of doing it himself. She also resisted all of our efforts to encourage Mr. Heller to push his own wheelchair from the bedside to the kitchen table for lunch, saying, "You don't know my husband like I do. He's just not strong enough." By doing that, she was not only undermining our care plan—she was undermining his self-esteem.

She treated her husband as if he were a child, even going so far as to refuse to let us put pajama bottoms on him. Dressing him only created more work for her, she told us, because he was occasionally incontinent of feces. Also, he could use

 Lottie insisted on taking total charge. She tried to control every aspect of her husband's home care. With her long, silver hair and squat, rugged body, she reminded us of a chunk of granite, indomitable and utterly self-contained. What she lacked in strength, she made up for in boundless determination.

the bedpan much more easily if he didn't have to take off his pants first.

If body language was a weapon, Lottie Heller had an arsenal at her disposal. Each morning after breakfast, as we gave Mr. Heller his bed bath, she'd stand by with her hand on her hip and her face contorted by a look of annoyance so deep and abiding you'd have thought she'd been born with it. And maybe she had. "Put the soap back in the

soap dish—don't let it set there in the water," she'd say, pointing a gnarled finger at one of us.

Unfortunately, her complaints weren't limited only to mornings. She expected us to return exactly on time for Mr. Heller's midday meal, and if we didn't, she'd be waiting in the doorway with her hand on her hip. "I told you to be here at 11 and no later," she said one day, glaring at us. "My husband's a diabetic, *in case you've forgotten,* and I can't get him fed on time if you don't get here until 11:30." One of us checked a watch. It read 11:02. That was Lottie's way.

But we weren't the only ones she was starting to wear down with her nagging. Week after week, as she nagged her husband, he became more and more an object of her control.

He'd ask her permission to use the bedpan, to eat, drink, or sleep. If he wanted to pull himself up by his overbed trapeze or just raise or lower his bed, he'd get her approval first. Lottie liked to watch afternoon soap operas and especially liked them *loud*—with the volume cranked up as high as their old Zenith would go. Once, we overheard Mr. Heller asking her to lower the volume so he could take a nap. She totally ignored him. The sound level stayed exactly where she'd set it.

Despite her psychological stranglehold on him, though, Mr. Heller's condition slowly improved. He still couldn't get out of bed on his own or even push his wheelchair from the bedroom to the kitchen. But by the second month of home care, he was continent of urine and feces and was having regular bowel movements. With weekly physical therapy, he could now raise one leg and then the other 2 feet (60 cm) above his bed while lying on his back. His incision line remained dry and intact.

If only Lottie's irrepressible behavior would show some improvement. To help us cope, we called in the agency social worker, who offered us some advice. We'll never forget what he said.

The ties that bind one family member to another—no matter if they are damaging or therapeutic ties—are generally much stronger than those that bind patients to their nurses. We couldn't expect to have any more influence on Mr. Heller than we were having already. Somehow, we had to change the way Lottie treated him by changing the way she treated us. You see, Lottie had built a castle around herself, her husband, and her home, and we were invaders, so she was suspicious of us and just about anything we did.

To strike a balance with Lottie, we agreed to follow three principles:

1. *Set priorities*. Was it really worth arguing whether the soap was kept in the soap dish or left floating in the basin water? If Lottie wanted it in the dish, we'd put it there. Similarly, if she wanted us to use corn starch instead of talcum powder on her husband, we'd acknowledge that her home remedy was just as effective.

On the other hand, we agreed that Mr. Heller must continue to try to push his own wheelchair to the kitchen every day—despite Lottie's strenuous objections—and that he should feed himself at the table.

2. *Be consistent*. Like many older people, Lottie was upset by the slightest change. So we decided to treat her husband as consistently as possible by meeting our daily schedule. We also agreed that each staff member would respect Lottie's idiosyncratic routines of care—as long as her methods didn't get in the way of proper nursing practices—and communicate them to all new staff members so they could follow them, too.

Finally, to make Lottie less suspicious of us, we rotated staff members only once a week.

3. *Don't overreact*. Getting angry at Lottie was easy. We recall the day we were orienting Susan, a new staff member. The afternoon before, we'd washed some of Lottie's laundry in town, folded it neatly, and placed it in her laundry basket. As we introduced Susan to Lottie, the older woman's eyes strayed to the basket, which we'd placed at her feet. Suddenly Lottie said, "Those clothes aren't folded right," and without another word, she picked up the basket and dumped it on the floor. The clothes spilled out in a tumble. After glaring at Susan, Lottie abruptly walked out of the room.

Susan looked shocked, and we felt like screaming at Lottie. But we held our tempers, picked up the laundry piece by piece, and folded it again. Later, when we were sure our anger had cooled, we looked for Lottie and found her alone in the kitchen. Only then did we learn why she'd acted the way she had.

She didn't say it outright, but her conversation showed that she saw Susan as another invader who would have to become part of their home life. That made Lottie uncomfortable. Very uncomfortable. By holding our tempers, we were able to get to the root of Lottie's childish behavior and understand her insecurity.

But believe us, unexpressed anger has a way of building up inside. To defuse these emotional bombs, the staff attended weekly sessions with the agency counselor. Those meetings were important in helping us stay relaxed so we could do our jobs better. Mostly we talked about Lottie and our efforts to change her. We soon nicknamed them "spill your guts" sessions.

Apparently, Mr. Heller had a lot of pent-up feelings, too. In time, he started talking back to his wife. Some days, we'd walk into a verbal firefight—their voices leaped through the tiny house like flames. He now *demanded* that the television sound be turned down when he slept. At first, Lottie only screamed back at him.

To referee their disagreements, we contacted our social worker again, and he agreed to give the couple counseling sessions. Also, we made a point of talking with them as a couple, rather than separately.

During those talks, we noticed something interesting. Mr. Heller would sit back and say just a few words before Lottie's voice swept him into complete silence.

Why? We wondered about that for awhile until we realized that he had difficulty recalling names, dates, and places. So to give him a fighting chance (verbally speaking), we'd intervene in conversations by making eye contact with him and asking, "What do *you* think, Mr. Heller?" Then we always waited for his reaction.

Our technique worked. Within a month, his powers of recall actually improved and his responses became quicker.

But despite all our entreaties, Lottie still refused to let her husband's bottom be clothed. We decided to call in Catherine, our director, because we knew she was the kind of woman Lottie respected—tactful but firm. We thought we'd never see it, but Lottie actually listened as Catherine explained that she expected Lottie to dress her husband the way he wanted.

Then, Catherine asked Mr. Heller how *he* felt about not being fully dressed, and he admitted it was humiliating. He was especially embarrassed when the neighborhood children looked in the windows and saw him. After their conversation, he smiled a smile we never saw before. It came flying right out at you like a rainbow.

The next day, Mr. Heller was wearing blue pinstripe pajama bottoms. What about Lottie? Well, it took her a week before she spoke to us again. We understood why, though. She was having a hard time accepting the fact that her husband was starting to declare his independence from her.

Spring comes to New England suddenly, as if someone just opened a heavy curtain over a picture window. And with the warmer weather Mr. Heller grew stronger. By April, he was getting around in his wheelchair with no help from us *or* Lottie. The decubitus ulcer had healed and his skin condition was excellent. His endurance was increasing—he could sit up for 4 hours straight. His favorite pastime now was to wheel himself outside on the porch and watch the local "foot people," as he called anybody traveling by foot along the road.

And how was Lottie coping with such a dramatic change? Well, the last few weeks had worked a tiny miracle. Some people try to be impregnable fortresses. But like a castle without an enemy in sight, Lottie had lowered her drawbridge a little to find she wasn't being attacked after all.

We didn't want to replace her loving attention. We only wanted to help her husband cope with his disabling illness. Lottie knew that, and she also knew something else. Now that Mr. Heller had become more independent and self-confident, he didn't need our care as much. We could gradually start phasing out our services. We thought she'd be pleased.

But perhaps she wasn't. One late afternoon as we drove away, we heard a voice and turned to see Lottie standing in the doorway. As usual, her hand was on her hip. But instead of glaring, she was waving to us. When she saw us looking, she quickly went inside the house.

Oh, Lottie. Maybe she'd never change—an 80-year-old habit is tough to break. But we could understand how far she'd come during the last few months. Slowly she was learning how to give a little.

Giving a little yourself is important when working with a patient's manipulative spouse. Generally, he or she meddles because of fear...fear of the spouse dying, of being left alone, or of any change at all. By treating the patient's spouse firmly but with compassion, you can cooperate to help make the patient's recovery smoother. It took a strong-willed mountain woman to teach us that.

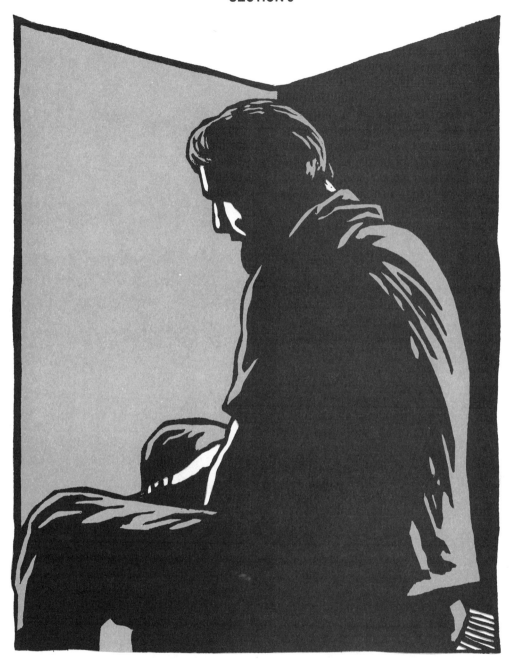

NONCOMMUNICATIVE PATIENTS

Drawing Robbie into a Circle of Love Just in Time

Sometimes, a patient's prognosis is so grim we know we can only provide supportive nursing skills, plus plenty of old-fashioned tender loving care. Suppose, though, the patient refuses that TLC? What can we offer then?

The same things, I'd say, plus a measure of acceptance and patience. But having cared for Robbie MacGregor, a desperately ill—and lonely—young boy, I guarantee you one nurse can't do it alone. Everyone involved with the patient must work together to create an atmosphere of caring.

Robbie, a 16-year-old victim of Ewing's sarcoma, had already undergone 2 years of chemotherapy when he was admitted to the oncology unit where I work. His oncologist wanted to check out a persistent sore on Robbie's upper lip and a disturbing increase in his white blood cell count.

Despite his youth, Robbie somehow reminded me of a battered, tired owl. Barely 5 feet tall, with spiky tufts of hair circling his head, he'd slouch down the hall, eyes cast down. When you'd speak to him, he'd look up, blinking large brown eyes made even larger by thick glasses.

Actually, he never gave us much chance to talk

to him. Even though his parents were his only visitors—and infrequent ones at that—he preferred to stay in his room, hiding behind a video game magazine or staring at the TV. When he did speak to us—usually to request something—he'd mumble, pulling nervously at the sore on his lip.

Robbie had every reason to be nervous: A bone marrow aspiration revealed that he had acute lymphocytic leukemia. We knew that meant more chemotherapy—and the complications that chemotherapy causes. What we didn't know was that Robbie would dare us to care for him.

Even the most independent teenager is usually glad to have his parents nearby when he's hospitalized. But Robbie insisted that we not let his parents in the room when we started I.V. infusions or other invasive procedures. "I don't want them to see me cry," he said. Yet he didn't hide his tears or complaints from us, virtual strangers.

Not that we wanted to stay strangers. But he responded to any offer to hold his hand during a procedure with a chilly, "Thanks, but no thanks." Worse yet, a comforting touch to his shoulder would bring a shudder. We could only stand, arms at our sides, not knowing how to comfort without being allowed to reach out.

Hoping to understand Robbie better, I watched his interaction with his parents, both Scottish immigrants. Mr. MacGregor was a quiet man who let his wife do all the talking. She'd insist, Robbie wants this or Robbie likes that. Mrs. MacGregor never really seemed to talk *to* Robbie, though— or even to her husband. The entire time I cared for Robbie, I never saw his parents touch.

Over the next few months, Robbie was repeatedly admitted to the unit, the stays lengthening each time. Those of us on the day shift gradually noticed that he was sleeping later in the morning. At first, we thought the extra sleep was just another way of avoiding us. During report, however, we learned that for several nights he'd been hanging around the nurses' station, talking into the early morning.

Thelma Moore, a night shift nurse, explained that one sleepless night had proved too long even

Robbie had every reason to be nervous: A bone marrow aspiration revealed that he had acute lymphocytic leukemia. We knew that meant more chemotherapy—and the complications that chemotherapy causes. What we didn't know was that Robbie would dare us to care for him.

for this determined loner. Around 11 p.m., he walked out to the nurses' station to ask Thelma to check his I.V. Then he asked her to fix his pillow, then to lower his shade…then to….

The mother of three teenagers herself, Thelma recognized the lonely heart behind the nervous chatter, pulled up a chair beside his bed, and did some serious listening. "All I did," she explained, "was ask if he'd ever played the video game *Frogger*. That got him started—he's always telling me about his video games now."

Encouraged by this breakthrough, we had a conference to talk about other ways of giving Robbie some companionship. One nurse suggested introducing him to Jennie, a 12-year-old girl recently diagnosed as having leukemia. That idea worked well. Pleased to play the role of the experienced older man, Robbie explained the ins and outs of chemotherapy to Jennie. The two quickly became friends.

Once Jennie was discharged, Robbie began to respond more to our friendly overtures. But he was obviously a novice at making friends. Finding our private lives nearly as interesting as his afternoon soap operas, he'd ask all sorts of questions: What were our husbands' or boyfriends' names, how many kids did we have, did we plan to have more, where did we go on vacation, how much would that cost anyway?

Most of us tried to be noncommittal in our answers—especially when he began to pass along information to our co-workers. With unusual insight, he probed into vulnerable areas, playing members of the staff against each other. Overweight or unattractive nurses were his favorite prey: "Mary Beth told me Annie's going to a dog show this weekend. No, wait a minute—I think she said Annie's going to be *in* it."

Cackling delightedly at his own jokes, Robbie apparently thought such sophomoric humor was his entrée into adult conversation. He didn't realize he was the only one laughing.

After discussing his barbs in a care conference, we made selective nonattention part of our nursing care plan. We simply wouldn't listen to disparaging remarks about colleagues. Once we presented a united front, consistently changing the subject to something more suitable, Robbie shelved his Don Rickles routine.

Because he had no friends his own age, Robbie tried very hard to identify with us. I can still see him pushing his I.V. pole down the hall, carefully making his way to the coffee pot at the nurses' station. Every day his hair seemed a little thinner, his shoulders rounder.

We'd pour him a cup of coffee and serve him his breakfast at a table just outside the station. He'd lean back and listen to our morning chatter. I can't remember him drinking that coffee, but there it sat beside him, a symbol of his adulthood.

After breakfast, Robbie sometimes asked if he could help us. Because his one hand had the I.V. line in place, we'd give him simple tasks he could do with the other—for example, ringing the bell to summon a nurse, stamping an Addressograph plate, handing someone a chart.

Once in a while, as we stood there talking while he worked, we'd forget and place a hand on his shoulder. He'd still shudder, though not so violently. He was learning.

Unfortunately, as Robbie became stronger emotionally, he grew weaker physically. The fevers started. His visits to the station became scarcer and shorter, then stopped. The sore on his lip grew and bled frequently.

Despite Robbie's poor condition, we tried to keep our budding relationship going. Several of us would join him in his room for coffee as we did our charting. We'd always ask, "Coffee'd out, Rob?" before we dumped his cold, untouched cup. His dignity was important to him. And to us.

His mother began coming more often and staying all day. At first we welcomed her visits; later, we dreaded them. I was shocked one morning to find Robbie actually begging for his breakfast tray as his mother calmly ate it in front of him. "No, Robbie," she said, "that poison's no good for you; take this drink instead. It's got lots of good vitamins. From now on I'll bring your food."

Every morning, Mrs. MacGregor arrived with a large thermos of megavitamin concoctions she called "health drinks." Every night, as soon as his mother left, Robbie prowled the halls, looking for food. Concerned, the night shift began bringing Robbie homemade stews and casseroles. When Mrs. MacGregor found out, she put an end to his nocturnal forages.

Robbie lost weight, his mother gained, as he drank the mega-vitamin concoctions, and she ate his hospital meals. Things came to a head one afternoon when Mrs. MacGregor slapped Robbie for refusing to drink his health drink. That slap

was the first touch I'd ever seen between mother and son. I suggested she go home for the day to rest; for once, she agreed.

When we told the oncologist we thought Mrs. MacGregor was becoming unbalanced, he asked the department social worker to talk to her. She reported that Mrs. MacGregor—who had at one time been under psychiatric care—was having

Finally discovering an opening to talk about his condition, I asked, "Rob, do you know what will happen if you quit trying?" "Yes," he said, closing his eyes. I let him rest. At the least, I was satisfied that he was aware of what was happening to him.

trouble accepting her son's condition. But the social worker cautioned us that since Mrs. MacGregor felt she should be at her son's side, we should respect her wishes.

We also had to respect her wishes about not discussing Robbie's poor prognosis with him. Although we'd offered our support and help in talking to Robbie about it, the MacGregors insisted that he'd be better off not knowing.

At this time, Robbie's oncologist suggested a new type of highly experimental chemotherapy. The MacGregors quickly agreed, but since no one asked Robbie, I did. He nodded okay, then said, through cracked and swollen lips, "If this one doesn't work, I don't want to try any more."

Finally discovering an opening to talk about his condition, I asked, "Rob, do you know what will happen if you quit trying?" "Yes," he said, closing his eyes. I let him rest. At the least, I was satisfied that he was aware of what was happening to him.

A few days later, Robbie's temperature soared to a startling 106° F. (41° C.). The cause? A possible fungal infection in his blood. We were to give him amphotericin B, an antifungal medication usually reserved for the most severe, hopeless cases—which described Robbie's situation all too well. After giving the first infusion, I waited to see what reaction, if any, Robbie would have. He screamed as the stomach pains began.

I reached for the meperidine (pethidine) I had ready to push in the alternate line and took his vital signs. Despite his acute pain, he was stable.

Mrs. MacGregor, who had watched the scene in horror, began crying hysterically. Another nurse came to my rescue: As she led Mrs. MacGregor away, she gently reminded her that this was an expected reaction and that we were already working to help him.

Soon we were giving Robbie some meperidine before and after each infusion of amphotericin B. Once, as I prepared to give him his next dose, his mother begged, "Hurry, give it to him, give it to him...he's going to die anyway. I'm so tired, I can't take it anymore. Let him die. When is he going to die...?"

I pushed the call light, and again, another nurse led Mrs. MacGregor out of Robbie's earshot. We pitied her then. She was trying hard to be a mother, but just didn't know how. Mr. MacGregor came to take her home.

For the rest of the day, we took up a vigil at Robbie's bedside, this time without the coffee. We knew he was too weak to notice.

The next morning, Mrs. MacGregor came back to sit—hardly moving—in a chair by Robbie's bed. She never spoke or touched him. I only hope he recognized the heartbroken love in her silence.

Robbie did let me know later that day that he recognized our concern for him. Since I couldn't be sure he'd be there on my return, I'd made a practice of stopping in his room at the end of my shift. As I stooped to kiss his forehead, he reached for my hand and squeezed it. I can't really describe the mixture of pleasure and sadness I felt. It was as if my heart were being squeezed, too....

Robbie died that night, holding Thelma's hand.

We had one last conference a few days later. For many of us, a sense of bitterness sharpened our grief: Why did someone so young have to die without ever knowing love?

"It's too late for Robbie now," I said.

"Was it really too late?" our unit coordinator asked. "You said he reached out to you, wanted to help you, held your hands. It seems to me you were just in time."

Perhaps she's right. I hope she's right. That all of us, working together and caring so much, had taught Robbie about love...just in time.

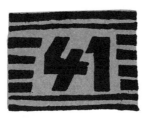

"Try to Keep Her Clothes on" Was the Staff's Only Goal

DEBBIE CASEY ROYALTY, RN, BSN

I was assigned to a state mental hospital for my student psychiatric rotation. There, for 7 weeks, I grappled with two problems: an anxiety-ridden patient, Betty, and an anxiety-ridden student nurse...me.

I was so unsure of myself that on the day I was to meet my assigned patient, I reviewed her history twice.

Betty was an obese, 67-year-old chronic schizophrenic. This was her fourth voluntary admission. On previous admissions, her diagnoses had also included manic-depressive psychoses associated with alcoholism.

Raised a strict Orthodox Jew, Betty had married at age 17 and converted to her Catholic husband's religion. She'd had three miscarriages and a stillbirth before her only child, a son, was born. The next year, Betty, at age 23, had a hysterectomy.

Her husband was an alcoholic "ladies' man." They were divorced but, some years later, remarried each other and lived together until the husband's death 5 years before.

Betty then moved in with her 40-year-old son and his 59-year-old wife. The fact that her daughter-in-law was only 3 years younger than Betty irritated her no end.

Betty, at 4'10" and 225 pounds, had been on an 1800-calorie reducing diet. I noted with surprise that, so far, she'd gained 5 pounds on the diet.

After I'd finished with the charts, I asked the charge nurse what kind of therapeutic relationship the nursing staff had established with Betty, and what special goals it was working toward.

"Look, just get her to keep her clothes on," she told me, "and you'll be ahead of the game." Then she walked off.

That was a blow. I'd been counting on getting some direction from the nursing care plan. Still, I couldn't postpone meeting my patient, so I went looking for her.

I located Betty rocking agitatedly in a rocking chair in the dayroom. (I soon found this was her favorite place.) She wrung her hands anxiously and constantly shuffled her feet back and forth on the floor.

I took a seat next to her. "Hi, Betty. How are you today?"

She looked at me and said, "Cox's army couldn't

keep them away. Taps is the loneliest sound in the world."

Then she made a loud, gutteral screaming sound, clenched her fist, and put it up to her mouth. I couldn't tell if she were trying to stifle the scream or about to strike me.

Fighting panic, I managed to say, "My name is Debbie, I'm a nursing student and I'll be working with you for the next 7 weeks."

"Congratulations, I crown you queen for a day," she replied.

At that point the nurse arrived. It was time for Betty to see her doctor. Greatly relieved, I told Betty I'd see her the next day, and made a hasty exit.

The next day I found her in the same rocking chair in the dayroom. When she saw me she said, "Oh look at that gorgeous creature. She'll have beautiful babies." All my prepared, introductory remarks flew out of my head as she went on and on about the day I'd fall in love, get married, and have beautiful babies. During the entire time I worked with Betty, she was obsessive about babies. Knowing her history of obstetric and gynecological problems helped me accept this.

Still talking about babies, Betty suddenly bolted out of her chair and disappeared down the hall. By the time I caught up with her, she was standing completely naked in the lavatory. The stalls had no doors and I saw feces all over Betty, all over her discarded dress, and all over the floor. I told her I'd help clean her up as soon as I went to the next room to get her a dress.

The hospital had a "community clothes box." Patients just picked what they wanted to wear from a few large boxes of used, worn clothing. By the time I'd found a dress I hoped would be large enough and had returned to the bathroom, Betty was standing in the shower with the water running. Now, there was feces all over the shower walls, as well. With no staff member either willing or able to help me, I cleaned up the bathroom and Betty by myself. When I finished, my clinical hours were over for the day and I had to return to seminar—with feces all over my clothes.

On my next care plan I identified "incontinent of stool" as one of Betty's major problems. She had only been incontinent once, but I was so anxious about my inability to form a relationship with the patient I misjudged it as a major problem.

After 3 weeks, I received a note from my instructor with the terrifying words: "Please see me."

I knew I needed to improve my approach to Betty and work out better care plans, but I didn't realize how poorly I was really doing. My instructor told me that she couldn't continue to accept such poor care plans. More important, I wasn't identifying any of Betty's real problems or needs.

Then the ultimatum: if there were no great improvement in the next few weeks in the way I was relating to Betty —and no improvement in my care plans—my instructor was sorry, but that would be the end of nursing for me. I just wasn't nurse material.

This has to be a nightmare, I thought. I'd wanted to be a nurse since sixth grade. *This couldn't be happening to me.*

That evening, I spent 3½ hours in my dormitory room analyzing my nurse-patient relationship with Betty.

Finally, I pinpointed the problem: I was taking her actions too personally. Whenever she was uncooperative or just ignored me, I took it as a personal rejection. I'd never before had trouble getting to know and get along with people. When Betty rejected me, I was just backing off out of hurt feelings... and a little hurt pride. This soul-searching helped me personally, but I had only 2 days to put together the first of my improved care plans. I decided I'd better attack a more obvious problem—Betty's obesity.

I understood its cause. Betty had told me her husband could never resist pretty women and he especially liked skinny ones. When he used to run around with them Betty would stay home and eat. "I feed everything I love," she said proudly. "The veterinarian told me I fed my dog to death."

That might explain her compulsion for food, but how could she be gaining on the hospital-regulated diet? The two obvious answers were: too many calories and too little exercise.

I began to observe her at meal times. Sure enough, Betty was eating off other patients' trays. When I sat with her during a meal, however, she was preoccupied with me and had no time to wander about sneaking food.

I arranged to have someone sit with her during

her other meals. I also persuaded her doctor to reduce her diet from 1800 calories a day to 1000.

That was the easy part. Getting her to exercise—even to move around—took more time. Because of obesity, Betty found walking a chore. The only trips she took were from the dayroom to the bathroom—a distance of 20 feet.

Not only would she not go to occupational therapy on the same floor, but she also usually "forgot" to go to the medication room. Then someone would bring her medicine to her.

The staff agreed to make Betty walk to the medication room for all her medications. At first, she was most resistant to this change. After I'd walked with her a number of days, though, she began going without having to be coaxed. Using the same approach, I also got her to go to O.T. twice a week.

The staff soon appointed Betty "errand girl" on the ward. Whenever they needed things like coffee cups and such, she would willingly go for them.

None of this increased activity caused her to lose weight, but at least she wasn't gaining any.

Searching for other simple, useful tasks, I began asking her to help me straighten the dayroom. This went pretty well. After a few days, I asked her if she'd get the dayroom in order (tables and chairs in place, ashtrays emptied) before I came. She agreed. After that, she'd point out how she was trying to keep the room neat.

I praised her to encourage her, and she seemed pleased. I was even more pleased. These worthwhile activities seemed to channel some of her anxiety. Her conversation rambled less. Often she would sensibly comment, "Well, I've told you that already, I don't want to bore you."

At this point, I timed her and found that she was able to stay on a reality-oriented subject for 1 to 2 minutes. *Finally*, I thought, *I'll be able to form a relationship with my patient.*

Each day, I began to ask Betty what she would like to talk about. I let her know I expected her to stay reality-oriented for at least 1 to 2 minutes. The fifth time I saw her after initiating this approach, she pleased and surprised me by asking agreeably, "Well, what do you want to talk about today?" What a pleasure to see that lessening of anxiety. That edging closer to normal behavior.

The next day I received another summons from my instructor. Suppose I hadn't measured up? Suppose my dreams of being a nurse were finished?

But I needn't have worried. The instructor told me that not only had my nursing care plans improved, but my approach to Betty had improved 100%. More significantly, she could see some improvement in Betty, herself.

Looking back on those 7 weeks, I see how I learned to write a good nursing care plan. And, because I experienced such tension and anxiety myself, I think I'll always be more empathetic with the anxiety in patients.

Possibly the most important thing that happened those 7 weeks, however, was the change in the staff's attitude. By the time my psychiatric rotation was over, they'd acknowledged the small successes I'd had with Betty. Building on my care plans, they established genuine therapeutic goals of their own for my patient—something more significant than, "trying to keep her clothes on."

Ms. Battersby...a Nurse Who Became a Demanding Patient

JANE BATTERSBY, RN

Stay away from 417! That message was as loud and clear as a fire siren. All you had to do was read the Kardex:

Rm. 417, Ms. B., 42-year-old female
Diagnosis—Sciatic pain
Up ad lib
Prednisone 5 mg q8h 8 am—4 pm—12 m
Valium 2 mg at bedside (qid or less as desired)
Patient makes repeated special demands.

These special demands as reported were:
1. Upon admittance, patient claimed the toilet seat had dried feces on it: wants it cleaned.
2. Repeatedly asks for extra pillows.
3. Declines to be awakened for 7 am temperature check.
4. Insists on walking to PT twice daily; refusing wheelchair, required by standing order for all patients going to PT.
5. Complained about another patient's behavior.
6. Demanded a patient-care conference with the supervisor!

That Ms. B. was some trouble, right?

Wrong. That Ms. B. *had* some trouble, which no one was concerned enough to try to correct.

And I speak with some authority because I am that "difficult patient," Ms. B.

I am also an RN and have heard, as often as you, that "nurses make the worst patients," an observation I would like to expand. It is truer, I think, to say that *anyone* who has a poor understanding of the nurse-patient relationship is likely to make a bad patient—and unquestionably a poor nurse.

It's been my experience, however, that the average nurse makes a better-than-average patient because she's seen both sides of the coin; she's "been there."

At the very least, the nurse will be in a better position than a layman to judge the quality of her care.

I am asking you then, as nurses, to judge the quality of care afforded this "difficult patient."

My initial hospitalization—before I was labeled the "difficult patient"—was a 3-day stay for tests. I had had chronic back pain for a number of years and my physician finally decided he wanted a workup. The spinogram proved negative—a circumstance that may later have influenced the staff to regard me as neurotic. (To keep the record straight, however, you should know that a year later, a more thorough test, a diskogram, revealed a degenerative process for which little can be done.)

During this initial hospitalization, I had received a Demerol injection into the right hip. The injection had made me wince and start with pain because the nurse had hit the bone. When I'd jumped, the nurse asked me if I was worried about something. I simply replied, "No, the injection hurt."

I was home from the hospital about 3 days when I started to experience such acute pain in the right hip and leg, I was unable to lift my leg and had to drag it to walk. I assumed that my problem was the result of the injection but when I called my physician he was reticent about discussing this possibility. He did, however, order me directly back into the hospital. There, he said he'd treat the periosteitis with rest, heat and cortisone and that the inflammation would probably subside in 10 days or 2 weeks. This was comforting, but I remained anxious. I couldn't help wonder if his curious uncommunicativeness was because of the gravity of my condition—or because he was afraid of incriminating the hospital.

Because I had such trouble walking and couldn't sit without excruciating pain. I was admitted on a litter to Room 417 by the admissions clerk at 4 p.m. The next person to enter my room was a nurse with a dinner tray. She placed it on the tray table out of reach and left the room. Since I was unable to sit up for dinner, I got up, got the tray and put it on my bed so I could eat lying down. When the tray was removed, I asked for a second pillow to support my painful leg. During the next 4 days I took complete care of myself, took my own shower, made my own bed and administered one of my two medications, which was kept at my bedside. Is that the profile of a difficult patient?

During this 4-day period, however, I did make requests… exactly four, not one of which was granted. They were:

"Please have someone clean the toilet seat in my bathroom."

"Please get me a second pillow."

"Please do not wake me at 7 a.m. to take a routine temperature." (I had no fever at any time—this was a local inflammation—and I knew the hospital had given up routine temps for most patients.)

"Please make a note on my Kardex that I walk to PT rather than use a wheelchair because I cannot tolerate the pain that results from sitting." (The chief physical therapist who had instituted the mandatory wheelchair rule understood my condition and also requested that I be allowed to walk to PT. Twice a day, however, someone appeared with a wheelchair, and we had this needless and wearing argument which, after much checking around, ended with my walking.)

The fact that I repeated these four requests a number of times brought no results at all, except that the repetition became "constant demands" in the eyes of the staff.

At the end of 4 days, I was distraught enough to ask to see the supervisor and to have a care conference in my room with her and the nurse in charge. The supervisor said she had never heard of a patient care conference with a *patient,* but agreed to do so. It was the first time I met the supervisor; the only other time I had seen the charge nurse was once when she had collected a lunch tray and we exchanged amenities.

During the conference, the supervisor's attitude was defensive and this is how the charge nurse answered my specific complaints:

1. The toilet seat was housekeeping's fault.

2. She would see that I got a second pillow.

3. She had 7 a.m. temps taken because otherwise one physician complained.

4. She did not know I could not sit without pain. (Although I had never told her this personally, I assumed she was in communication with her staff, who had been told repeatedly.)

The outcome of this conference appeared to be two-fold. First, I did receive the second pillow— 19 hours later… second, from then on, the charge nurse and supervisor resolutely avoided Room 417.

The morning after the conference, I was astounded to hear my physician confront me with: "I understand you were complaining about the woman in the next room." I had to think a minute before I recognized this as a distorted version of what had happened. Late at night, when a patient had become confused and wandered into my room, I had helped her back to bed. I then turned on my call light thinking surely the staff would want to know if a patient becomes confused and wanders about.

This, then, was a third effect of the conference—I was to be labeled a "difficult patient."

Instead of the interest and support of the nursing staff which I so desperately needed, I next received two public-relations visits from the director of nursing, who said that the administrator would pay my bill—a pointless gesture since I was covered by medical insurance. She further offered to send a TV to my room, but since this was something I preferred not to have, I declined. It arrived that afternoon.

This not-so-amusing comedy of errors made me analyze the situation from a nursing point of view. How does a perceptive nurse deal with a difficult patient?

First, she must ask:

Is this really a demanding patient? In my case, I had made exactly four requests before asking for the care conference. That hardly constitutes a demanding patient. However, these requests *were* made repeatedly.

That's when the nurse must ask:

Are these requests legitimate? If they are, then she must find out why they are being ignored and make it her responsibility to honor them.

The concerned nurse will try to pierce the aura of mutual misunderstanding that usually surrounds a "difficult patient."

She will ask:

Is it the patient or the situation that is difficult? In this case, fear of a lawsuit over the badly-placed injection during the first hospitalization influenced the staff's attitude, I'm sure. Although I had no intention of suing, the presence of that possibility made for a "difficult situation," made the staff anxious, and provided them with excuse enough for ignoring me. All difficulties considered, however, surely even a difficult patient is still entitled to minimum nursing care.

Possibly the most important question the knowledgeable nurse asks is:

Are staff and patient really communicating? The good nurse recognizes the difference between a pleasant conversational encounter and a patient-nurse communication. In my case, during a genuine conversational exchange I could have discussed my legitimate fear of possible loss of the use of my leg. Nurse to nurse, we might also have explored my concern over a possible cortisone reaction. At the very least, we could have gotten my needs registered on the Kardex. But there was never such an opportunity.

And, quite clearly, the staff members were not communicating among themselves. If they were, the wearing, twice-daily misunderstanding about the wheelchair would have been avoided; the charge that I had complained about another patient would never have occurred.

But it did. And I was the "difficult patient," sick—and afraid—among nurses who avoided me. It was a very lonely experience and need never have happened if we had just been able to communicate.

Communication—that is the clue that was missing in this entire situation—right up to the end. And so, you won't be surprised to learn that on the day that I left, the feces was still on the toilet seat... I was given a bill for the TV... and they brought a wheelchair to discharge me!

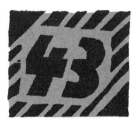

Mr. Ming Gets the Message

FRANCES STORLIE, RN, MS

Have you ever had a "difficult patient" who was really a dear?

It could happen, you know, because sometimes the difficulty of the situation has nothing to do with the personality of the patient.

That's how it was with Ming Lam.

Mr. Lam, as we first called him, was a Chinese merchant seaman who suffered an acute inferior infarction while his ship was docked in Portland, Oregon. When I first saw him in the coronary care unit, he had sinus tachycardia and frequent, multifocal premature ventricular contractions. His face and manner were stoic, and his hands were calmly folded across his chest. But I thought I saw fear in his eyes. Of course, I could have been projecting my own feelings. I had once been sick in the strangeness of Chicago, and was really afraid.

In the first hours, we did the usual things for Ming Lam... started an IV of Xylocaine, called a cardiologist, took an EKG, and gave him a pain medication on the orders of the resident. And oh, how we would have liked to reassure him—at least explain what was happening to him. But Ming Lam's entire English vocabulary consisted of the word, "okay"—which put him one up on us because we didn't know any of his language.

We put in a call to Nursing Service, asking them to search out people who spoke Chinese. Our hospital had no formal list of staff members who speak a foreign language (most large hospitals would find one useful). But we hoped that in our 500-bed hospital we might find several persons of Chinese descent.

Meanwhile, we had to deal with Mr. Lam as best we could. After he'd been in the unit a few hours, we agreed that he *must* want a urinal. The nurse took it into him, pointed to the approximate position on herself where one might be placed, then handed it to Mr. Lam. Twenty minutes later, we still hadn't heard from him—so the nurse retrieved it. It had been used. This proof that sign language works encouraged us to try something else. We drew a picture of a heart in a body which was wired to a monitor. Then using this, we pointed to his wiring and to the monitor on the wall behind him. But this time we were pretty sure he didn't understand our meaning. Or did he?

Speech experts tell us that over 20,000 difficult

facial expressions are somatically possible. During that first difficult period, I think our nursing staff must have touched base with all possible combinations to convey their feelings of reassurance, encouragement and friendly concern.

Nursing Service finally located four staff members who spoke Chinese, but only one nurse spoke Ming Lam's dialect, Cantonese. She came in from another floor and explained some of the novelties of hospital living—like the use of the call light. She told him what the cardiologist had said about his heart; she demonstrated the connection between the wires and the monitor and promised to come back to talk whenever she chould. She also told us that since the Chinese place the last name first, we couldn't be calling him Mr. Lam, but Mr. Ming!

On his second morning in the CCU, we saw evidence that Mr. Ming hadn't understood all that had been explained—at least not about the call light. While watching several patients from the central nursing station, I suddenly saw Mr. Ming retching. He had already stopped vomiting by the time I got to his bedside. He handed me the urinal. I smiled and started out when I was aware of his excitement. He pointed frantically to his mouth then to the urinal. I shook the receptacle and, sure enough, his dentures rattled away in the vomitus. "Okay, I'll get them," I gestured into and out of the mouth of the urinal. After I thoroughly cleaned and replaced the dentures in his mouth, he smiled slightly and said, "okay, okay." I hesitated on the brink of trying a conversation—but what was okay, the teeth, my nursing action? Or did he feel better, less nauseated?

Pausing at the door, I noticed him watching me intently. "Okay," I said and with my thumb and index finger made the round "okay" sign. Then I left. I didn't realize that Mr. Ming would take that gesture to mean goodbye until I saw him use the sign every time anyone went out through his door. Finally, a puzzled doctor asked me about this, and I found myself explaining rather lamely, "Well, meanings are whatever two people agree they are. Ming Lam and I know what we mean."

We asked the interpreter to teach us a few Chinese words of the "Hello, how are you" variety but Ming Lam never spoke Chinese to us. He would parrot exactly what we had just said in English. He learned the essentials—"hungry"... "toilet chair"... "no pain"... "water"... "go home," (by this, we assumed he meant that he wanted to), and, of course, "okay." So mostly, we found ourselves chattering away in English to Mr. Ming in exactly the same way we did to our other patients. After all, language expert S. I. Hayakawa maintains that the purpose of "small talk" is not to communicate information but to establish communion. And prevention of silence is itself an important function of speech. In our dealings with Mr. Ming, I think this theory was well proved.

Whenever we had to make important changes in treatment, however—like discontinuing the IV, increasing his exercises, transferring him to the progressive cardiac unit—we made sure we had interpreters on hand to explain the changes to him. And, because someone who is sick and apprehensive often forgets things that were explained just a few minutes before, we asked the interpreter to write down the explanation and leave it on the bed stand so Mr. Ming could refer to it when he wished.

Mr. Ming's ship had already sailed back to China, and he received exactly one visit from the steamship line's representative. It was a helpful visit because Mr. Ming learned that his wife knew of his attack, recovery, and anticipated return within a few weeks. But it didn't seem enough. A heart attack is a major life experience—for some, the last. And it is fraught with uncertainties regardless of how much support is given. So we sent out a call for more interpreters to visit. One of our lab technicians and his sister, a college student, came faithfully. Although they couldn't speak his dialect, they could write in Chinese, which he understood.

Hoping to communicate with Mr. Ming in another way, one of the nurses brought in a bouquet of red and white asters. Surely, the gift of flowers is universal, we thought. But Mr. Ming just touched them and looked puzzled. Only later did we learn that in the Orient, fruit or cake are the ordinary gifts for the convalescent. And in the Chinese culture, red is a symbol of joy and white for mourning. No wonder Mr. Ming looked puzzled!

One thing there was no mistaking was Mr. Ming's desire to please. "Okay, okay" remained his favorite phrase. Still there must have been times when it was very difficult for him. One morning when I found him staring at the ceiling, breakfast untouched, I tried to think of something universal and simple we could share. I borrowed snapshots of another nurse's small children and took them to Ming Lam.

"You got children?" I asked.

"Got children," he said. "Two. Two children."

I continued, "Boy or girl?"

"Boy and girl," he answered.

He handed back the pictures and I started to leave the room. "Aha, making headway," I thought.

Suddenly he was talking again, "Seven. Seven children," he finished.

I will never know whether he has two children, seven children, or seven grandchildren. Or maybe two children by a first wife and seven by a second? I also wondered if the conversation had helped him—or possibly depressed him further by making him homesick for his family.

Another morning when he seemed down, we called the interpreter and told her we wanted to treat Mr. Ming to a telephone call home. It would cost less than 75 cents for each of us; the time in Canton was checked and the steps for putting a call through to China were initiated. At this point, the interpreter wisely interrupted, "Does his family have a phone?"

She engaged Mr. Ming in conversation and I watched his face light up with pleasure and finally he laughed. It was the first time we'd ever heard him laugh.

"He says they have no telephones where he lives but you are so nice nurses—very good and nice."

Later when we discussed this case, there were some things that seemed left undone. We regretted not having thought of calling an Oriental church or hospitality center—or even a seaman's institute—in search of possible visitors for Ming Lam. And we had noticed that Ming Lam received much less sedation than we generally administer for infarction, reflecting his insistence that he had "no pen, no pen," whenever nurses or doctors so much as touched or pointed to his chest. But did he have no pain? Wouldn't admitting to it likely keep him in a strange land and away from his family longer? These are things we'll never know.

After 3 weeks in the hospital, Ming Lam was scheduled to fly home, and we celebrated with a chocolate angel food cake with whipped cream frosting. How alone Ming Lam looked seated at his bedside table with the cake, fork and napkin in hand.

"How's the cake?" someone asked. I was standing at the door as she began to exit from the room. Ming Lam made the okay with thumb and forefinger. The nurse looked at me and we both laughed. "Okay, or goodbye?" she asked me.

It didn't matter in the least. Words aren't the only way to say "we care" and I think Ming Lam got the message.

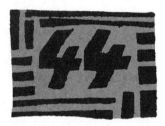

Lisa and the 2 O'Clock Miracle

LORRAINE M. LYNN, RN

Like most nurses, we psychiatric nurses try not to use medical jargon around patients. We know the risk of being misunderstood. But some psychiatric patients, living in a world of their own, are so unreachable we can't communicate with them no matter *what* kind of language we use. Twenty-two-year-old Lisa Carson was such a patient.

When I arrived at work the day after Lisa's admission, the atmosphere on the unit seemed tense. As I passed the observation room, I heard a loud humming and a thrashing sound. I peered through the window and got my first glimpse of Lisa. She was restrained in a Posey vest and was rocking back and forth, her eyes clamped shut, her hands folded as if in prayer. Even from a distance I could see she was covered with sweat.

At morning report, I learned that Lisa would be my patient, so the other nurses filled me in on the details of her admission. The morning before, Lisa's mother had brought her into the emergency room. Lisa was covered with cuts and bruises, her feet were swollen, and she was filthy. She was also completely out of touch with reality.

According to Mrs. Carson, Lisa had left for beautician's school the morning before but hadn't returned that night. Worried, Mrs. Carson had called the police to report her missing.

Then at 3 a.m. Mrs. Carson had received a call from an elderly couple in a nearby city. They'd seen Lisa staggering around the street and had taken her in. She was incoherent, but they'd found identification in her purse. As they were making the call, however, Lisa had slipped out and disappeared.

At 7 a.m., she'd limped barefoot through the door of her house. From the looks of her, she'd walked the whole way home—about 20 miles.

Mrs. Carson had told the nurses she didn't know what'd happened to Lisa. Up until 2 years before, she'd been "a good girl who did what she was told." Then Lisa had begun acting "strange," and after her father died of a heart attack, she'd gotten stranger still.

The nurses told me that Lisa's behavior was so disruptive and bizarre the other patients were afraid of her. She'd been on the unit only 1 day, but so far she'd run down the hall naked, defecated on the floor of her room, urinated in her bed, and tried to wash her hair in the toilet. She repeated ritualistic arm movements, and when any of the other patients tried to talk to her, she'd kneel on the floor and kiss their shoes. Finally, the nurses had restrained Lisa, for her sake as well as the other patients'.

The doctors started Lisa on large doses of thiothixene hydrochloride (Navane) and amobarbital (Amytal), but she continued to be extremely agitated. Until the doctors found the right combination of drugs to control her behavior, we knew any—except the most basic—nursing interventions would be futile. So for the time being, we resigned ourselves to just being Lisa's caretakers.

By the end of that week, the drugs began having a tranquilizing effect on Lisa, but the side effects were worrisome. She twisted her head sharply in one direction while she rolled her eyes in the opposite direction. She drooled and moved her legs and feet randomly. Her doctor took her off Navane and put her on haloperidol (Haldol). The day after Lisa began taking Haldol, we witnessed the "two o'clock miracle"—as it came to be known—for the first time.

I entered Lisa's room that day, and for once, she was resting peacefully. But the odor of urine and sweat was overpowering. We'd been keeping her door closed to protect her from the curious stares of visitors and other patients, and her room was like a stinking sauna.

Wishing I didn't have to inhale, I took Lisa's hand in mine and said, "Hi, how're you feeling?" We weren't sure if she understood us, but we always talked to her as if she did.

To my amazement, Lisa answered, "Hello/who/are/you?" Her eyes remained closed, and her speech was machine gun rapid, but for the first time, she'd responded appropriately.

"I'm Lorraine, your nurse," I said. "Why don't you open your eyes and see what I look like?" Lisa opened her eyes, struggling to focus on my face.

"Lorraine/Lorraine," she said in a monotone. "The/rain/in/Spain/falls/mainly/on/the/plain/that's/how/I'll/remember/Lorraine."

Looking at Lisa, I tried to imagine what she'd been like before. Her mother said Lisa had been *fastidious*—bathing several times a day, changing her clothes just as often. Now, Lisa looked a mess,

despite our efforts to keep her neat.

She sure could use a shower, I thought. But when I suggested a shower to Lisa, she pleaded, "Oh/no/please/oh/no/please."

Knowing that *I'd* probably get a shower, too, I stripped to my underwear. Then I undressed Lisa and put her under the shower. She continued to protest, but when I used too much shampoo on her hair and we got covered in bubbles, she turned her face toward the shower stream and smiled beatifically.

I dressed Lisa in jeans and a T-shirt, sat her in a chair near the nurses' station, and began to feed her. We'd tried letting her feed herself, but her ritualistic arm movements made this impossible. This time, whenever Lisa began moving her arms, I put a piece of fruit in her hand and firmly instructed her to eat. She did.

When Lisa had finished eating, I tuned the unit's radio in to a rock station, and Lisa sang along, perfectly in tune. While she sang, I brushed her long blond hair and caught it in two ponytails. Everyone remarked on how nice she looked, and she beamed happily.

Then Lisa began slipping back into her own world. She stopped singing and began humming tonelessly. And she started rocking and moving her arms randomly. I gave her her medication and then returned her to bed, restraining her once again.

After that, we witnessed the two o'clock miracle every day—although it wasn't always at 2 p.m., sometimes it was at 4 a.m. Nevertheless, Lisa remained in the real world for about 2 hours every day, and even though we couldn't keep her from slipping back into that other place, we were content that she was sleeping soundly and perspiring normally. Small accomplishments, for sure, but not to us.

Since we were never certain when the miracle would occur, we never knew how Lisa would be when we entered her room. One day, I found her standing naked in the middle of the floor, rummaging through a paper bag.

Oh dear, I thought. But when I asked her what she was doing, she answered appropriately. "Looking for my deodorant. My aunt's coming to visit and I want to freshen up."

When I asked Lisa how she was feeling, she

said, "Better, but I'm still a little shaky. I guess it's all the medicine."

Lisa's speech was still quite rapid, but she wasn't speaking in a monotone anymore, and her responses seemed appropriate.

The doctors were as encouraged as we were by Lisa's daily periods of lucidity. But they felt that

 We witnessed the two o'clock miracle every day—although it wasn't always at 2 p.m., sometimes it was at 4 a.m. Nevertheless, Lisa remained in the real world for about 2 hours every day, even though we couldn't keep her from slipping back into that other place...

these periods were too brief, and the possible side effects of the drugs too risky, to continue with our present treatment. At best, we were maintaining Lisa in a borderline psychotic state. The doctors wanted to try electroconvulsive therapy (ECT), and under considerable duress, Mrs. Carson agreed.

Lisa had her first ECT a few days later, at 7 a.m. After the treatment, I walked her slowly back to her room and helped her into bed so she could nap.

When I checked on her at 8:30, she was just starting to wake up. "Hi, do I know you?" she said sleepily. "Don't you remember 'Lorraine and rain in Spain'?" I asked hopefully. But she didn't, so I reintroduced myself.

The doctors began giving Lisa a new sleeping medication, along with the ECT and the tranquilizers. Although she was still somewhat agitated during the day, she was lucid for longer and

longer periods. The two o'clock miracle was, at last, stretching out over most of the day.

I'd been Lisa's caretaker for 2 weeks when she finally improved enough that I could start one-to-one therapy. Now that she was coherent much of the time, I hoped I could help her put her confused feelings into words. I also hoped that when she started hallucinating, I could lead her back to reality.

During our first therapy session, Lisa paced nervously around the room. "I don't know why I do this," she said. "I know I'm acting crazy."

I assured her she wasn't acting crazy—she was just letting off steam. But Lisa's fear of being labeled "crazy" was obvious. So I was careful not to use psychological terms with her, although sometimes I found myself groping for substitutes.

One word I found a *very* effective substitute for was "hallucinating." Whenever Lisa started slipping out of reality, I'd ask, "Are you watching home movies again?" She took my words in good humor, and more often than not, she snapped out of her hallucination—at least temporarily. And since no stigma is attached to watching home movies, she was often able to talk about her hallucinations in a straightforward way.

Lisa also talked about her family. At first, she had only nice things to say, but her facial expressions belied her words—especially when she talked about her mother. Then, her face registered anger and something very close to hate.

I wanted Lisa to get in touch with her real feelings and then respond appropriately, so I held a mirror up to her face. She was amazed at what she saw. Eventually, as she grew to trust me more, I'd interrupt her in midsentence, hold up the mirror, and then ask her to repeat what she'd just said.

Finally, Lisa admitted to herself and to me that she *hated* her mother for criticizing her and making her feel ugly and stupid. Lisa felt that even though her mother visited often, she did it only for the sake of appearance.

Over the next few days, Lisa told me more and more about her family. Both of her parents had been rigid disciplinarians and strict churchgoers. Mrs. Carson repeatedly warned against getting "too friendly" with boys, and consequently, Lisa'd never had a boyfriend for more than a few weeks.

Then, Lisa told me she blamed herself for her

father's death. Her mother said she "broke her father's heart" because of her craziness.

After Lisa told me her story, she didn't need to look in the mirror so often, so I put it on the bedside table. Occasionally, Lisa'd pick it up and examine her face when she talked. But eventually, she stopped using the mirror altogether. She asked me to leave it on her table, though, because to her, it'd become a symbol of "realness."

Besides our one-to-one sessions, Lisa began going to daily patient discussion groups and participating in unit activities. We encouraged her to be more assertive, and the other patients gave her support. They told her how good she looked and how smart she was. One woman patient returned after a weekend pass and presented Lisa with a pretty, little ring. "When you look at this ring, remember that we love you," she said. Lisa told her she'd never take it off.

As Lisa became less withdrawn, she became more interested in her appearance and wanted to lose the several pounds she'd gained during her hospitalization. We encouraged her to diet and helped her select low-calorie foods. Lisa spent a lot of her restless energy washing and slicing raw vegetables, and since many of the other patients also had weight problems, she enlisted their help, too. Soon kitchen duty became a real social event.

After a month on our unit, the doctors felt Lisa was well enough for discharge. She would, of course, continue drug therapy and see a psychiatrist regularly.

The last time I saw Lisa, I'd just begun working the evening shift, and I was supervising a patient party in the lounge. To everyone's amazement, one of our most withdrawn patients suddenly picked up a guitar and began to sing in a beautiful, clear voice. All the patients and staff gathered around, singing along. Lisa looked especially happy. She seemed to be off in a private world, but from the look on her face, it was a peaceful world—not at all like the place she'd once retreated to.

She was having such a good time, I didn't have the heart to interrupt her to say goodnight—and good-bye. But when I reached the door, Lisa ran up to me and hugged and kissed me. "I'm having such a good time tonight," she said happily. "This is appropriate behavior, isn't it, Lorraine?"

And it *was*. Behaving appropriately may not seem like much of an accomplishment to most people, but to Lisa, it was her ticket back to the real world.

Reach Out, Reach Out and Touch…Henry

CHRISTINE MAREK, RN, BSN

We live in such a highly verbal society, we sometimes overlook other forms of communication. When I need reminding, I think of Henry, a patient on whom all our verbal skills were useless.

When Henry arrived at our orthopedic unit on a stretcher, he was waving his arms frantically and yelling incoherently at the top of his booming voice. He was in pain and badly frightened. His strength and vigor made it hard to believe he was 80 years old. He'd fallen and suffered a displaced subcapital fracture of his left hip, but that wasn't the only thing that had sent him into a panic. Henry had been blind and deaf for close to 40 years and had lived in the same nursing home for almost 20 years. He had no idea where he was or what was happening.

For the time being, we restrained Henry as best we could while moving him from his stretcher to a bed. Then, the orthopedic resident applied Buck's extension traction to Henry's left leg. We medicated Henry with meperidine (pethidine), 50 mg intramuscularly, which seemed to relieve his pain, but there wasn't much we could do about his anxiety and disorientation. As a result, he constantly squirmed around in bed, defeating the purpose of the traction. When we found him with both legs dangling over one of the side rails, we realized he simply could not safely be left where he was. We had little choice but to put him in a net bed. This left him some movement and a modicum of control over his situation.

It wasn't hard to understand Henry's fears. Here he was in a strange place, physically confined, surrounded by unfamiliar people doing things to him that he didn't really understand. How would we ever orient our patient to the new environment and make him realize we were there to keep him safe and help him get well?

The primary nurse soon realized that Henry relied heavily on his sense of touch to understand incoming messages. He liked to have his hand held and his shoulder patted, and he settled down noticeably whenever he felt a gentle touch. After a while, he even became confident enough to lie still and talk quietly.

Soon we all learned to touch Henry's hand whenever we entered his room.

"Hello," he'd say. "I'm glad to see you."

Patting his arm before he got an injection or rubbing his shoulder after any procedure clearly meant a lot to him.

"I'm better now," he told us. "Thanks for taking care of me."

As Henry relaxed (and peace and quiet returned to the unit), everyone became a lot less frustrated. We realized, however, that it was going to take more than a touch on the hand or a pat on the shoulder to prepare Henry emotionally for his upcoming surgery. Why, we couldn't even tell him he was going to have surgery. Nonetheless, every attempt was made to establish a trusting relationship.

Henry's son came as often as he could. Henry did recognize him and was obviously reassured by his presence. Since this was about the only familiar connection Henry could make in this completely unfamiliar environment, we encouraged the son's visits.

Henry was taken to surgery for a hip arthroplasty with an Austin-Moore prosthesis. He tolerated the procedure well and returned to the unit 4 hours later.

His postoperative care presented a whole new set of challenges. At our hospital, a patient with an Austin-Moore prosthesis can be turned for very brief periods, but most of the time he has to lie with a pillow between his legs. This position prevents dislocation of the prosthesis. How Henry's stayed in place I'll never know, since he shifted position so often.

Fortunately, Henry was allowed out of bed the day after surgery, and this gave us a way to channel some of his energy. So with two people helping, Henry pivoted out of his bed and into a reclining chair.

"Thank you," he said. "This is nice." Then he sat quietly for a couple of hours. It certainly was nice.

Henry didn't seem to understand why he had a bandage on his left hip, and he was determined to get it off. Furthermore, as soon as he got the dressing off, he'd go to work on his staples. We just couldn't allow this, so we reluctantly put mitts on his hands. We took them off for baths and meals so Henry could at least help with his own daily care and retain some measure of self-sufficiency.

On the whole, Henry progressed well through his postoperative course. We kept him oriented with a regular, consistent routine of daily care. After the first day, he always sat up in a chair for meals and rested in bed in between.

On his fifth postoperative day, it was time for Henry to try to walk. With one nurse on each side, he stood and walked about 20 feet. The only problem was that he would sometimes sit down without

 It wasn't hard to understand Henry's fears. Here he was in a strange place, physically confined, surrounded by unfamiliar people doing things to him that he didn't really understand. How would we ever make him realize we were there to keep him safe and help him get well?

any warning at all. We solved that one by having a nurse walk behind us with a wheelchair ready to catch him whenever he decided to sit. After a while, with daily help from a physical therapist, Henry was able to get around with a walker and a single nurse as a guide.

Henry's wound remained free of infection and began to heal nicely. His staples were removed, and 2 weeks after admission, he was returned to his nursing home.

We were really pleased with Henry's progress and proud of ourselves for being able to return him to his previous level of activity. Unfortunately, we were a little premature.

Three weeks later, Henry fell again and had to be readmitted. X-rays showed that the Austin-Moore prosthesis was in place, but the wound had dehisced.

Once again we faced the challenge of keeping his incision free of infection. This time, however, the wound was open, and our job was a lot harder. Every 8 hours, we irrigated his hip with half-strength peroxide followed by normal saline solution. Then we packed the wound with iodoform gauze. To do this, we had to turn Henry onto his unaffected side and put two pillows between his legs. He wept with pain the first time we did it. Hoping to make him more comfortable the next time we irrigated him, we administered pain medication a half hour before the procedure. Unfortunately, there was no way to tell Henry that this irrigation was going to be any easier than the last one. He fought us as hard as he could, yelling "Leave me alone. You're going to hurt me."

It took several of us to get Henry through those first few irrigation procedures. He never understood why we were probing and packing his wound, but he did begin to realize that it wouldn't hurt. Each time we'd hold his hand and turn him as gently as we could. Someone would rub his shoulder while we irrigated and packed. When we finished, we'd always stay a couple of extra minutes just holding his hand. It doesn't sound like much, but it worked. After a few sessions, Henry tolerated his irrigations well and even turned over for us by himself.

He never accepted his dressing, however. Even with mitts on his hands, he could get his bandage off and pull the packing out the minute your back was turned. In time, purulent drainage, cultured as *Staphylococcus aureus,* began oozing from the wound. So a regimen of intravenous antibiotics was added to the regular irrigations. After a week, the drainage was serosanguineous, but the wound showed no signs of healing. Henry's doctor, worried that the hip might be infected, ordered exploratory surgery.

Fortunately, there was no infection. The fascia was debrided and the wound closed with wires. A skin graft was considered, but in order for a graft to live, it can't be disturbed. The patient must remain immobilized for several days. Obviously, Henry was not a good candidate. The wires would have to do. With mitted hands and close supervision, Henry left them alone. We irrigated the wound every shift with half-strength Dakin's solution and packed it with a normal saline wet-to-dry fluff gauze dressing. This had to be inserted through the wires, and the whole procedure was pretty time consuming. Blessedly, the wound soon began to show evidence of granulation.

By this time, Henry was quite at home with the hospital environment and routines. He seemed to understand why we were there and began to communicate his needs and affections freely. A far cry from the panicky, thrashing patient who'd arrived, he remained friendly, cooperative, and grateful. After 2 months, he returned to his nursing home, his wound completely healed and free of infection.

Henry's course was a complicated and sometimes frustrating one, but his special problems taught us the enormous value of touch as a means of communication.

To Communicate with Mrs. Savage, We Put Bells on Her Toes

CAROL E. SCHREIBER, RN

Every nurse has known at least one patient who needs constant care. Mrs. Savage couldn't see, she couldn't speak, and she couldn't move anything except her feet. With Mrs. Savage, we bent over backward to make her well.

Forty-three-year-old Mrs. Savage was admitted to our hospital with blurred vision and bilateral ptosis. Within 24 hours, she developed respiratory distress and generalized weakness, and was transferred to the intensive care unit (ICU), where an emergency tracheostomy was performed and she was put on a ventilator.

The next day, her weakness had become paralysis, which affected everything but her feet. Her spinal fluid showed increased protein, and a diagnosis of Guillain-Barré syndrome was made.

We thought we knew a lot about caring for Guillain-Barré patients—we'd had several in the last year. But Mrs. Savage wasn't a typical Guillain-Barré patient. Instead of ascending, as we expected, her paralysis had descended, affecting her optic nerves. Although her eyes were always slightly open, her vision was so blurred that communicating with alphabet boards or flash cards was out of the question.

But Mrs. Savage had her own way of communicating. Every time we approached her bed, she'd wiggle her feet wildly. Obviously, the disease hadn't affected her hearing, and she seemed totally alert. But when she wasn't moving her feet, she looked like a corpse.

We put Mrs. Savage in the bed closest to the nurses' station and checked on her every 10 minutes. We assured her that people with her disease *do* get well, and that soon she'd be able to see again, to speak, to move, and to breathe without a ventilator.

Our first job was finding a way to communicate with Mrs. Savage, and, since none of us had ESP, we knew we'd have to learn foot language. We thought, *If we make her right foot the "yes" foot, and her left foot the "no" foot, we can ask her questions and she can answer us.* But first, she needed a way to get our attention.

I bought a string of Indian brass bells, and using umbilical tape, fastened one bell to each of her feet. The ringing was loud enough to be heard easily, even in the din of the ICU.

Talking with bells wasn't easy, and sometimes we asked Mrs. Savage questions for an hour before pinpointing her problems. Eyes burning? Earache? Headache? Suctioning? and on and on until we got a "yes." Mrs. Savage even had a signal for "erase and start over"—she'd ring both bells simultaneously.

Mrs. Savage was a pathetic sight, and she looked worse with each passing day. Her mouth hung flaccidly open, almost down to her chest, and she

 Our first job was finding a way to communicate with Mrs. Savage, and, since none of us had ESP, we knew we'd have to learn foot language. I bought a string of Indian brass bells and, using umbilical tape, fastened one bell to each of her feet. The ringing was loud enough to be heard easily, even in the din of the ICU.

drooled constantly. Her dentures wouldn't stay in place, so we removed them. Her hair began to turn gray and fall out. She was pale and flabby.

Our nursing care plan for Mrs. Savage was simple—we simply did *everything* for her. We put an alternating pressure mattress on her bed and turned her every 2 hours to prevent pressure sores. We applied antiembolism stockings to her legs to prevent phlebitis, and dressed her in high-topped sneakers (4 hours on, 2 hours off) to prevent foot drop.

We did passive range-of-motion exercises on every joint of her body, including her jaw, several times a day. Three times a day, we lifted her out of bed, ventilator and all, and sat her in a high-backed chair for a half hour. We restrained her in the chair with seat belts, propped up her arms on pillows, and tied up her jaw with a chin strap.

Then came the beauty treatments. We turned Mrs. Savage's room into a regular Elizabeth Arden salon. While she sat in the chair, we soaked her feet, and then did pedicures. We manicured and polished her fingernails. (They'd been bitten down to the quick when she was admitted, but now they'd grown fashionably long.) We washed and set her hair, and shaved her legs. Do you know we even dyed her hospital gowns bright colors and told her how nice she looked. We knew that when she could see again, she'd appreciate what we did for her.

The ICU was filled to capacity that summer, but somehow we still managed all this extra care for Mrs. Savage. To help her feel secure, the same nurses cared for her all the time. We read to her and told her the news and weather. We brought her a radio and a tape recorder with talking books. And we waited anxiously for signs of improvement.

Mrs. Savage's vision began to improve first. After 4 weeks in the ICU, she was able to open her eyes halfway, though still not far enough to read flash cards. And she still couldn't close her eyes completely, so that when she slept, her eyes looked like slits. But we were so encouraged by this small improvement, that we put her glasses on her every time she sat in the chair.

Shortly after her vision improved, Mrs. Savage was scheduled to have a feeding gastrostomy tube inserted under local anesthesia. We didn't anticipate any problems—we felt we'd built up a surprisingly good rapport with our patient. But when we explained the operation to her, Mrs. Savage rang her bells in what seemed like terror. We realized then how dependent on us she'd become. We assured her she'd be able to talk to the operating room staff with her bells, but as she was wheeled out of the room, she shook her "no" bell frantically.

The gastrostomy tube was inserted, and, thankfully, Mrs. Savage calmed down and adjusted well to the tube. We all felt relieved—until she developed earaches. She was barely over her ear problem when she got pneumonia. Although we knew pneumonia was a common complication for a patient who's on a ventilator for any length of time, we still felt discouraged.

With antibiotics, Mrs. Savage's pneumonia cleared up, and we resumed our routine of lifting her into the chair. Except for the slight improvement in her vision, Mrs. Savage's condition remained the same.

We relaxed the visiting rules so Mrs. Savage could have visitors at all hours of the day. Her husband came every day and read her books and magazine articles. He called her Tinkerbell, and he and Mrs. Savage "talked" about everything from her flower garden to the latest neighborhood gossip. They even had a few arguments—like the time Mr. Savage admitted he'd forgotten to water the houseplants and they'd died. (Mrs. Savage rang her "no" bell until we thought her foot would fall off.)

After 8 weeks in the ICU, Mrs. Savage complained of leg pain. In spite of our constant exercising, and the antiembolism stockings, she'd developed phlebitis. Until the phlebitis improved,

"Try, Mrs. Savage, try!" we coaxed, as we unhooked the ventilator. She panicked, ringing her bells wildly. "You can do it," we assured her. Then she'd hyperventilate until we hooked her back up.

Mrs. Savage had to stay in bed. Apparently annoyed that she wasn't getting her full schedule of beauty treatments, she began ringing her bells constantly. But when we'd run down our list of questions, she'd "erase" every last one.

Some days we wanted to throw her bells in the trashcan. The doctors were getting short-tempered, too. Mrs. Savage's chart became more and more unwieldy, and every time a doctor opened it, papers fell on the floor.

We grew increasingly suspicious that Mrs. Savage had ambivalent feelings about getting better. Yes, she wanted to get better and return to her life of being a housewife and a nightshift factory worker. On the other hand, she resisted our efforts to get her to resume responsibilities that would hasten that return.

For example, Mrs. Savage's eyesight had improved enough for her to read flash cards, but when we propped up a book in front of her, she flatly refused to read. She still wanted us to read to her. And even though she could now move her eyes to answer us, she insisted on using her bells. Clearly, she was afraid we'd take away her bells.

When her phlebitis improved, we sat her in the chair again, and tied her bells to her knees instead of her feet. But she wouldn't try to move her knees. She'd just glare at us with her eyes almost popping out of her head.

Eventually, we were ready to wean Mrs. Savage from the ventilator, regardless of whether *she* thought she was ready. So we started disconnecting the ventilator every time we moved her to the chair, always explaining what we were doing, reassuring her, and making small talk. As long as she was distracted, she could breathe on her own without panicking.

"Try, Mrs. Savage, try!" we coaxed, as we unhooked the ventilator. She panicked, ringing her bells wildly. "You can do it," we assured her. Then she'd hyperventilate until we hooked her back up.

We asked for a psychiatric consultation. (By this time, we nurses needed one too.) The psychiatrist believed that Mrs. Savage thought we were lying to her about being able to breathe unassisted. We, however, suspected that Mrs. Savage was intent on controlling us. After many weeks of coaxing and prompting, Mrs. Savage took a few breaths on her own and began to swallow her saliva. We praised her lavishly. A few more days of coaxing, and we had her off the ventilator and breathing on her own for the first time in 4 months. While she breathed, we *held* our breath. After 2 weeks off the ventilator, we knew she'd finally made it.

To prepare her for transfer to a medical floor,

we took her for wheelchair rides to her new floor. We introduced her to the nurses and wheeled her into her new room. At first, she panicked, but then her panic seemed to turn to anger. She wouldn't even look at us.

Five months after her admission. Mrs. Savage was transferred to the medical floor. Now, *we* were panicky. *Suppose she regressed again?* But she didn't—she adjusted. Although her arms and legs were still flaccid, she began to move her head and jaw. Her gastrostomy tube was removed, and she began eating baby food.

Then her tracheostomy tube was removed, and she began going for physical therapy. We visited her several times a week, encouraging her to try to talk. She ignored us.

One day, a nurse on the medical floor called to say that Mrs. Savage had started talking. We were elated. My first free minute, I went to see her.

I thought excitedly, *Now she'll be able to tell me what we could've done to make things easier for her, so next time we get a "Mrs. Savage" we'll give even better care.* I admit I also anticipated her thanking us for the loving attention we'd given her.

But when I got to her room, ready for a long chat, she looked at me, and in a whispery voice said, "I don't want to talk to you. You're not my nurse anymore." On the brink of tears, I left her room.

When other ICU nurses visited Mrs. Savage, they met with the same reaction. Her nurses on the medical floor said she never chatted with them, either. She only made demands. Six months after her admission, Mrs. Savage was discharged to a rehabilitation hospital.

A year after her discharge from our hospital, I saw Mrs. Savage in the supermarket. I hardly recognized her. Her hair had grown back, she was stylishly dressed, her false teeth were in, and her nails were still long and well manicured. This time she spoke to me, saying that she was returning to work soon. Except for a slight weakness in her right arm, she looked like any other housewife. In fact, she looked better than most.

Perhaps we'd expected too much from Mrs. Savage. Wanting your patient to try to get well is one thing, but expecting her to be grateful is something else entirely. In her own way, Mrs. Savage probably *was* grateful, but her gratitude shouldn't have been so important to us. The important thing was that we'd made her well again. And judging from the way she looked, our beauty treatments had given her a new pride in herself. When I saw her that day, I knew we'd done right by her. And certainly in one way—by recovering and looking so well—Mrs. Savage had done right by us, too.

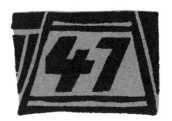

When We Tried to Get Close to Carrie, She Pushed Us Away

MARY ELLEN REBELE, RN, BSN

If all our patients were textbook cases, none of them would be difficult. We'd simply look up the directions on how to care for "patient A" and get perfect results every time. Of course, no patient ever conforms to a textbook description. Twelve-year-old Carrie Johnston was dying, and according to the books, she should've been progressing toward the acceptance stage. But Carrie hadn't read the books—she was *mad* at what had happened to her. And every time we tried to get close to her, she pushed us away.

Nine months before, when Carrie'd first been admitted to our pediatric unit, she'd been bouncy and talkative, jabbering about music, horses, and school. She'd been admitted because of slurred speech, weakness on her right side, and difficulty walking. A computerized axial tomography (CAT) scan had revealed a metastatic brain tumor, and in surgery, the doctors found they would never be able to remove it all.

After surgery, Carrie, who was started on cobalt and steroid therapy, seemed angry and depressed most of the time. But who could blame her? She was old enough to know that something was very wrong, yet the doctor had advised the Johnstons to postpone telling her that, at best, she had a year to live.

For some months after her discharge, Carrie did quite well. She worked hard to keep up with her studies at home and tried to help her mother around the house. But when she began having severe abdominal pain and difficulty swallowing, she was readmitted to our unit.

Even though I've cared for other patients with brain tumors, I was shocked by Carrie's appearance. Most of the hair that'd been shaved before surgery had grown back, but it'd changed from flaxen to dirty blonde. Her face was moon-shaped and puffy from the cortisone therapy, and her once-petite figure was gone—she'd gained 25 pounds (11.4 kg).

Carrie and I had been good friends during her first admission, and I'd hoped we'd pick up where we'd left off. But when I tried to take her hand in mine, she pushed it away and turned her back to me. *Why, she seems more angry and depressed than 9 months ago*, I thought. *I wonder if she's been told she's dying?*

When we were alone, Mrs. Johnston told me that she and her husband *had* told Carrie about her prognosis. And Carrie's reaction had been violent. She'd screamed at them, accusing them of lying. As if to prove to herself and her parents that she *wasn't* dying, she began studying extra hard and talking constantly about returning to school.

The Johnstons were despondent. Over the months, *they'd* learned to accept their daughter's death, heartbreaking as it was. But Carrie's reaction to any mention of her prognosis was so violent, that helping her seemed more than difficult—it seemed impossible.

After talking with Mrs. Johnston, I called a staff conference. Our first priority, of course, was to make Carrie trust us enough to confide in us. Only then could we help her learn to accept her coming death. But Carrie had a long way to go and a tragically short time to get there. Her second admission would probably be her last. We hoped if we were patient and loving enough, Carrie'd respond.

But the more patient and loving we were, the more hostile Carrie was. Her speech became more slurred every day, and we had to listen extra carefully to understand her. Still, when we said, "You can talk to us, Carrie, about anything that's bothering you—it's all right to be angry, you know," she'd respond by pointing her finger toward the door. We didn't have any trouble understanding *that* signal.

When Carrie was admitted the first time, she knew little about sickness and hospitals. By her second admission, she was an expert. She knew all the nursing procedures by heart and fought us during most of them. She shook her head violently when we approached with the bath tray, pulled away when we tried to take her temperature or other vital signs, and became frustrated when we didn't put her on the bedpan in exactly the position she wanted. She never seemed to enjoy her wheelchair trips around the unit and seemed relieved when we returned her to bed.

Carrie continued to have trouble swallowing and, eventually, couldn't even tolerate a liquid diet. So the doctor inserted a gastrostomy tube. Since she was only 12 years old, the mere *idea* of a tube entering her stomach embarrassed her. But the *sight* of the tube actually horrified her. We took

great pains explaining the procedure, trying to make it as acceptable as possible.

Naturally, we were meticulous about her gastrostomy care—placing a linen saver over her bottom sheet and watching carefully for any backflow of liquid. If any of the feedings did accidentally soil her bedclothes, Carrie's embarrassment and horror turned into rage—at us.

When we changed her dressings—a procedure she found especially repulsive—we always pulled

 Our first priority, of course, was to make Carrie trust us enough to confide in us. Only then could we help her learn to accept her coming death. But Carrie had a long way to go and a tragically short time to get there.

the curtain for extra privacy, even though she had a private room. And we tried to get the procedure over with as quickly as possible. But nothing satisfied her.

Beneath Carrie's hostility, another, stronger emotion began to grow—fear. She was afraid that in her sleep, she'd choke to death on her own saliva. She insisted on having her bed elevated at an 80-degree angle at all times. And she fought sleep fiercely.

True, Carrie *did* have trouble swallowing, but her problem wasn't as serious as she imagined. Hoping she'd sleep longer, we administered her tube feedings and checked her vital signs at 6-hour intervals during the night. But she continued to lie awake most of the night.

Because of her fear of choking, Carrie insisted that one of her parents be at her bedside constantly. Since her father was a truck driver and on the road most of the time, the responsibility fell to her mother. And the poor woman was almost asleep on her feet. If she left the room for even a few minutes, Carrie'd call out in panic and threaten to pull out her I.V.

Obviously, our care plan wasn't working. Carrie'd been our patient for 3 weeks, and she still wouldn't even talk to us, although we did everything we could to earn her trust. When she rang her call bell, we ran to her room in a flash—hoping our eagerness would convince her of how much we wanted to help her. When she made threats, like saying she'd pull out her I.V. anytime her mother left, we'd just remind her that her mother needed a break but that *we'd* stay with her until her mother returned. Carrie usually responded by turning her back to us.

I recommended that a nurse thanatologist be brought in, but my request came too late. By then, Carrie's right hand was so weak she couldn't write, and her speech was so slurred even her mother had trouble understanding her. More to the point, we doubted Carrie would've accepted a new nurse. She barely tolerated *us*.

Carrie was denying her death just as vehemently as the day she'd arrived, and nothing we did seemed to have the slightest effect. Then, out of desperation, we came up with the idea of a "sunshine box" filled with gifts to be opened, one each day. We knew that sunshine boxes worked with younger children, but with Carrie?

Then we thought, *what 12-year-old (or adult, for that matter) doesn't love opening presents?* We passed the word around to the staff, asking them if they'd like to contribute. We covered a cardboard box with colorful circus animals and wrote a note to Carrie expressing our affection. In a few days, the box was filled with pretty, wrapped packages— perfume, jewelry, stuffed animals, nightgowns.

When we carried the box into Carrie's room, we weren't sure what kind of reception we'd get. We hoped she wouldn't turn her back or point to the door. And she didn't. She was genuinely surprised, and for the first time since her admission, she smiled.

She chose the biggest present first and playfully put the pink bow on her head as she opened the box. Inside was a soft, flannel nightgown from one of the nurse's aides. When we asked if she'd like to wear

the gown, she said she'd rather wait until morning, when she'd had her bath and shampoo.

This was the first time Carrie'd shown an interest in her appearance, and we were elated. Each time she opened a new present, she opened up a little more to us. Each day, she chose her gift for the following day and then asked the nurse who'd contributed the gift to be in her room when she opened it. She stopped refusing her morning baths and was even willing to spend short periods of time alone. It was almost too good to be true— the box of gifts had brought the sunshine back to Carrie's face.

Although she never told us in words, we thought Carrie'd finally realized that we cared for her as a person; that we didn't consider her just another problem patient. We'd been trying to tell her precisely that for 3 weeks, but a simple gesture like a sunshine box had broken through her wall of anger and depression. We thought: *Perhaps actions do speak louder than words*.

Although Carrie's emotional health seemed greatly improved, her physical health was deteriorating. She still had persistent abdominal pain of referred neurologic origin. She asked for pain medication more frequently, but the meperidine (Demerol) the doctor prescribed made her constipated, depressed, and irritable. So the doctor decreased the amount of Demerol, increased the time between doses, and prescribed diphenhydramine (Benadryl) to help her relax. Carrie adjusted well.

Carrie was also beginning to adjust to the gastrostomy tube—its appearance didn't seem to bother her as much as before. Unfortunately, though, she wasn't adjusting well to the feedings, and her stomach was painfully bloated most of the time. We asked the doctor if he might decrease the amount of solution and the length of time between feedings, and he agreed. This alleviated much of the pain and bloating. As more time passed, Carrie began to show an interest in her tube feedings, asking us what different kinds of fluids she could have and joking about wanting a milk shake through her tube.

Although she still insisted on keeping her bed elevated, she was sleeping soundly. For some reason, she needed less suctioning and actually seemed to be growing stronger. One night, she asked if she could do her own suctioning, and I helped her use a hard-tip catheter. Then she asked if she could try drinking some juice. We experimented with several kinds of oral fluids, but I had to suction out most of them. Carrie wasn't discouraged though—she hadn't tasted anything for so long, she was obviously enjoying the sensation regardless of the suctioning. After we finished, she pointed to the intake and output sheet, indicating that she wanted me to record the amount of fluid she'd taken by mouth.

I was so encouraged by Carrie's sudden progress that I asked the doctor if he thought we should begin discharge planning. He cautioned me that her progress was probably only temporary, but he encouraged me to discuss Carrie's possible discharge with her parents. Since my shift was ending, I decided to talk to them the next evening.

But when I walked into Carrie's room the next evening, I knew instantly that something was wrong. The sunshine had gone from her eyes, and in its place, I saw fear.

"You feeling okay, honey?" I said. And then Carrie did something she'd never done once in the 5 weeks I'd cared for her—she reached out and grabbed my hand. Worried, I pulled a chair close and tried to discern what was different about her.

The skin on her right side looked mottled, as if something was wrong with her circulation; her breathing seemed labored; and her chest sounded congested.

Then, Carrie threw her arms around my neck and said, in a voice I could barely understand, "I'm scared, Mary Ellen." I held her close and rocked her, telling her not to be scared, that we'd take care of her. When I felt she was comfortable, I told her I was going to get her parents, but one of the other nurses would stay with her until we got back. I immediately summoned the Johnstons and the doctor, because I knew Carrie was dying. Two hours later, wrapped in her mother's arms, Carrie quietly died. The doctor took no heroic measures.

Looking back, I think that even though she'd never discussed it openly, Carrie had come to accept her death. It seemed that somewhere between opening her first gift and opening her last, she'd stopped being angry; stopped denying. That last night, when she tried so hard to take part in her care, I think she was rewarding us for all *our* weeks of caring. How could she have known that just seeing the sunshine in her face again was all the reward we'd ever need?

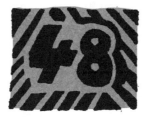

Mr. Peters Was Afraid to Face Me… and His Problem

MARY ANN GREGG, RN, BA

Have you ever been assigned a patient you couldn't even get to meet? Well, I have, and after enough unanswered letters, ignored phone messages, and unkept appointments, I'm tempted to close the file and write him off as "an unresponsive patient."

Looked at in another way, however, such a patient *is* responding. And very often, the message he's sending is: "I'm too frightened and depressed to face you… or my problems." Can we in conscience close our ears to such a message?

Mr. Peters was a 53-year-old bachelor whose only family consisted of a married sister who lived 700 miles away. He worked as a credit manager of a lumber yard where, 2 years before, he'd stepped on a nail. The puncture had become infected and, in being treated, he learned for the first time that he had diabetes. Gangrene set in, and his right leg below his knee had to be amputated.

Mr. Peters was fitted with a prosthesis and attempted to return to work. He had, however, acquired the poor walking technique of stomping on his left foot to spare pressure on the right stump. This caused a grade IV diabetic plantar ulcer to develop on his left foot. So, in an effort to save his foot, he was sent to a nursing center for intensive nursing care. Mr. Peters was in the center only a few days when a diabetic retina hemorrhage caused the loss of vision in one eye.

Three months later, as a rehabilitation specialist, I was assigned to help Mr. Peters formulate goals for rehabilitation and eventual return to normal life.

I sent a letter explaining this goal to Mr. Peters and asking him to choose a day when I could see him. I included stationery and a stamped return envelope for his convenience. When I didn't hear from him in 2 weeks, I called the head nurse. She knew about my letter and told me that Mr. Peters said he didn't want to see me.

In my experience with uncooperative patients, I've found that if I can just gain the confidence and support of the people around the patient, that relationship will sometimes serve as a bridge to the patient himself. I asked the head nurse to tell me everything she could about Mr. Peters. She did, and ended the lengthy discussion by urging me to try to get through to Mr. Peters because he needed help.

I told her to tell him that I'd be in the center the next week and perhaps we could get together then. The next week, however, he still refused to see me. Respecting his decision, I didn't enter his room, but I did leave my card and a handwritten note telling him I'd call again perhaps when he felt better.

So that my visit wouldn't be a waste of time, I met with Mr. Peter's occupational and physical therapists and the dietician. They gave me further insights to my elusive patient. Without ever getting to meet him, I was starting to know Mr. Peters a bit.

The first break in what seemed to be an impasse came that night. I got a call from a Mr. Wilson, who roomed in the same boarding house as Mr. Peters. He said the patient had asked him to call me and assure me that he didn't want to see me.

Now that might not sound like much of a break, but look at it this way: it was the first time *Mr. Peters* had initiated the contact.

I asked Mr. Wilson to assure Mr. Peters that I had no intention of forcing him into anything. I just wanted to talk to him. Then, with a little questioning, I got Mr. Wilson to fill me further in on Mr. Peters. I learned that Mr. Peters was "down in the dumps. His friends have mostly forgotten him. He's given up... won't get out of bed or shave or take care of himself." Mr. Wilson ended by saying he hoped I *would* get to talk to Mr. Peters.

In contrast to the patient's stated position, I felt I was getting a lot of messages that he *did* want to see me. But I knew I mustn't crowd him.

I took no action for 1 week. I wanted Mr. Peters to think about what I meant when I spoke of rehabilitation. I also wanted him to wonder if I had taken him at his word and written him off.

At the end of the week, I called the head nurse again and asked her to tell Mr. Peters that I'd be at the center on Tuesday and Wednesday and ask him what time would be convenient for him. I planned this approach to assure him that I respected his independence as a person. He could still refuse to see me. If he would see me, however, it would always be on the day and hour of his designation.

The message came back: Mr. Peters was *not* interested in any rehabilitation. But he would see me.

On Tuesday at 10 a.m., we finally met. All the background information I'd been collecting over the weeks made the meeting much smoother. I was prepared for the unshaven, messy-looking, clearly depressed man lying in the bed. I was already knowledgeable about his physical, personal, and occupational problems.

He, in turn, must have been thinking a good deal about this meeting, too, because he really opened up. Here was a man who'd had seven operations in the past 2 years. He'd lost one foot and was threatened with loss of the other. He'd lost the vision in one eye and was worried about the second. He had no close family, few friends and, as a 53-year-old mentally competent man, found himself confined to a nursing home, watching the end of life flicker from the aged and senile patients around him. We never mentioned the word rehabilitation, but its very first requirement, getting the patient to express his feelings, had been fulfilled.

To preserve the feeling that I was *not* pressuring Mr. Peters, I continued using the head nurse as intermediary. She'd tell him what days I'd be in the center. He could decide if he wanted to see me. The second time we met, I told Mr. Peters I'd contacted both his internist who was treating the diabetes and his orthopedic surgeon who was waging the fight to save Mr. Peters' left leg. This gave Mr. Peters the opening to discuss his unspoken fears.

He'd been off his foot for 4 months now, but the plantar ulcer hadn't yet healed. He was afraid it never would. I assured him the doctors believed it would.

He'd lost 20 pounds since the fitting for the first prosthesis. A poor-fitting prosthesis would throw his walk off and cause the ulcer to reopen. I told him he would be refitted.

But even if he were discharged, where could he go? How could he live alone? How could he learn to shop and cook for a diabetic diet?

This recitation of these genuine anxieties was an encouraging sign. It showed me that Mr. Peters believed enough in the possibility of rehabilitation to be worried about it.

Before I left, I asked him if he was restricted

to bedrest. He admitted that he was allowed in a wheelchair as long as his leg was elevated but he just never had the ambition. I made no further comment.

I waited 2 weeks before contacting him again. This time I found Mr. Peters not only shaven and neat looking, but in a wheelchair socializing with other patients. Clearly his self-identity was returning and, along with it, his confidence and hope. He chided me for not having contacted him the week before. He asked the nurse to change the dressing on the ulcer while I was there so the three of us could discuss its status.

Before I left, he confided that Mr. Wilson and he were considering getting an apartment together and splitting the expenses. I told him how pleased I was that he was making plans because doctors' reports suggested that his discharge was definitely coming. This was a significant meeting because it was Mr. Peters who initiated the tentative plan for living with Mr. Wilson. This proved to me that the patient had accepted rehabilitation as a reality.

He now used the phone at the nurses' station to make appointments with me. He asked me to be his luncheon guest at the center. And he bore up under the inevitable reverses. A nurse, for example, in changing the ulcer dressing, pulled off some skin. With the decreased circulation, diabetes and months of slow healing, the tape burn was a depressing setback.

Another time, an orderly dropped Mr. Peters' ulcerated foot while showering him, causing the ulcer to separate and bleed again. These problems were overcome, however, and finally he was walking with only a cane.

Mr. Peters was fitted with a new prosthesis and began spending trial weekends in his new apart-ment with Mr. Wilson. During those last few weeks in the center, we saw that Mr. Peters got intensive teaching on the importance of hygiene, urine testing, diet, and food preparation. Four months after his initial refusal to see me, the man who didn't want to be rehabilitated was discharged.

Yet, this was not the end of all problems. His prosthesis was not completely right and had to be refitted. The living patterns of two confirmed bachelors were too different to be reconciled, and Mr. Wilson moved out. Mr. Peters was hospitalized twice for scrotal abscesses. Still, he did not despair. Together we assessed the problems as they arose and worked out their solutions. Mr. Peters is currently job-hunting and has had two encouraging interviews.

Working with this patient has proved to be one of my most rewarding experiences. It's been a pleasure to watch the nurse-patient relationship develop from a 100% effort (all on my part) to an honest give-and-take between two people.

Mr. Peters, for example, who's come to like cooking, experiments with diabetic exchanges to improve various recipes. I try them on my family, and they enjoy them. He entered my name for a free subscription to the *Diabetic News* because he thought I'd appreciate it, and I do. The night his doctor was speaking at a conference in town, Mr. Peters notified me because he thought I'd like to attend. And I did. All this from the man whose file I could have closed 10 months ago because he was "an unresponsive patient!"

The one thing we're still looking forward to is his return to productive employment. Then, I'll happily close Mr. Peters' file... this time with the notation "rehabilitation services completed."

When It Came to Communicating Without Words, Cyrus Was an Expert

SUSAN RAMAGE PRESLEY, RN

Sometimes conventional problems call for very unconventional solutions. I'm thinking of Cyrus, who was our patient a year ago.

Cyrus, a 67-year-old retired farmer, had been admitted to an outlying hospital with a diagnosis of chronic obstructive pulmonary disease with end-stage emphysema, inactive tuberculosis, and pneumonia. He'd been intubated, supported on a ventilator, and tracheotomized. But when repeated attempts at ventilator weaning failed and his secretions became unmanageable, he was transferred to our coronary care unit. He weighed only 85 pounds (38.3 kg) and was gray as a ghost. An almost constant stream of thick, green sputum erupted from his tracheostomy.

Laboratory tests showed that Cyrus was malnourished, so he needed a nasogastric tube for continuous Isocal feedings and I.V. fluids to correct electrolyte imbalances. Amid all the equipment, the small man looked buried. Also suspicious. And scared. In the beginning, Cyrus seemed almost totally alienated from his surroundings.

He was alienated from us, too, because he couldn't talk. But he refused to try any of the usual methods of nonverbal communication, like an alphabet board or flash cards. And he was too weak and uncoordinated to write anything we could read. He insisted on using pantomime to "talk," and we tried hard to understand his gestures. But the harder we tried, the more annoyed Cyrus got. He'd dismiss us with an exasperated, defeated grimace and a wave of his skinny hand. And when his wife couldn't understand him, he'd dismiss her in the same way.

We had to admit, though, that Cyrus's body language *could* be effective. Before long, he'd developed a unique way of calling us—he'd simply pull his tracheostomy tube out of the ventilator tubing, triggering a loud alarm. By doing this, he got a double point across—"I want you in my room *now*" and "I hate this ventilator."

Frankly, Cyrus's physical care was often downright messy. We had to suction him at least every 30 minutes, and when we disconnected him from the ventilator, his cough sent sputum flying in all directions—on him, on us, onto his tracheostomy dressing, and 6 inches (15 cm) up the ventilator tubing. His care was also tedious because besides the suctioning every half hour, we also repositioned him frequently to prevent decubitus ulcers and contractures. With all these interruptions and his almost constant coughing, Cyrus got little sleep.

We couldn't blame Cyrus for being in a bad mood—who wouldn't be? Still, we felt frustrated and inadequate. Although Cyrus's care took a lot of time, it wasn't that complicated, and we knew we could help him if he'd only let us. We decided that we might be able to earn his trust if we created more continuity in his care. So a few of us volunteered to care for him several days in a row if we were relieved of our other duties on those days.

Cyrus responded well to our new care plan, and during the next week, things began looking up. We got him out of bed and into a chair several times a day, and he started having physical therapy. With the increase in activity, he slept better. He also began taking small oral feedings, although Isocal was still his main source of nourishment. We suggested that his physical therapy sessions be spaced so he wouldn't get too tired before mealtimes, and his therapists agreed.

And then the big breakthrough came. Cyrus's doctor ordered that the tracheostomy cuff be deflated and the stoma plugged every 15 minutes so Cyrus could talk. We weren't surprised when one of the first things he said was, "I can't live like this. Get me off this ventilator."

For 2 glorious days, Cyrus talked. He asked questions about his illness and treatments, and we tried to explain everything to him in layman's terms. As his mood improved, he became more cooperative and even began eating more.

But then we suctioned soft food from Cyrus's tracheostomy when the cuff was deflated. Fearing that he'd choke, we switched him back to full liquids and kept his cuff inflated at all times. We tried to make him understand why this was necessary, but he wouldn't accept our explanations. Because Cyrus couldn't talk anymore, he was furious.

He didn't have any way of expressing his anger. He couldn't scream, was too weak to kick, and was too uncoordinated to even write curses on paper. He needed to release his anger somehow. So we tried our first unconventional idea—we gave him a rubber-shod hemostat and told him to bang on the bedrails whenever he felt angry or needed

something. Within a half hour, he was banging all the time. And by the end of the shift, we were ready to lynch the nurse who'd first suggested giving Cyrus the hemostat. But we endured the racket—if banging on his bedrails would help, we'd learn to cope with the noise.

Then we began to see a pattern in Cyrus's behavior. Because he'd lost all control over his situation, he began making demands that would help him feel in charge.

He called us—via hemostat—all the time. Then, using mime, he'd remind us that we'd been late in feeding him or turning him, and he'd demand

 Because Cyrus couldn't talk anymore, he was furious. He didn't have any way of expressing his anger. He couldn't scream, was too weak to kick, and was too uncoordinated even to write curses on paper.

to know exactly what time some part of his care would be done. He began making demands on his family, too, insisting that his wife or one of his three married children visit every day. For them, this meant driving 125 miles (200 km), often over icy, hazardous roads. But they did it. We relaxed the visiting rules for them and let them bring things like posters, cartoons, a cassette player, and a radio to keep Cyrus's spirits up. But even that wasn't enough.

One icy night, after Cyrus's wife had returned home from the hospital, he demanded to see her again—no particular reason, he just wanted to see her. To pacify Cyrus, we called his wife. Over the phone, we interpreted his pantomimes to her. We later used this method on several occasions when bad weather prevented his family from visiting.

Cyrus's demands soon extended to a meticulous structuring of his environment. We'd moved him into a larger room, partly to accommodate the growing collection of greeting cards and posters that covered the walls and partly to keep an eye on him. His new room was within view of the control monitor consoles, where one of us was always stationed. Having a nurse always in sight calmed Cyrus, lessening the number of times he summoned us. He even gave up bedrail banging for a civilized call light.

But everything in his new room had to be just so. His urinal belonged on the bedrail, his bedpan under the sheet within his reach, his facial tissues on the bed outside the sheet, and his wastebasket on the floor near his bed, where he could easily drop tissues into it. We all complied with these "rules"—after all, they were small concessions to make if they made him feel more in control.

By this time, Cyrus had made considerable progress in communicating. He had a regular repertoire of mimes, including "bed up," "bed down," "urinal," and "doctor." One of his more dramatic renditions was "the room is too hot," for which he'd fan his face and hang his tongue out of his mouth. We helped each other interpret these mimes and passed the information on to his respiratory and physical therapists. When we couldn't understand one of his mimes, Cyrus would make a writing sign. Now when we gave him a pen and paper, he could write a few legible words.

His doctor increased his Isocal intake from 1,500 to 2,000 ml a day. Things seemed to be going well, and he was gaining weight. We began removing the ventilator when he coughed, allowing him to expectorate into tissues. Then one day we discovered that he was coughing up green-colored Isocal through his tracheostomy. A bronchoscopy showed that the Isocal was being refluxed from his larynx into his trachea. Obviously, Cyrus's Isocal intake was more than he could handle.

But he still needed a high-caloric intake, so we discussed with him the possibility of removing the nasogastric tube and inserting a jejunostomy tube. Cyrus refused to permit this, insisting that he could eat enough by mouth. We knew he couldn't possibly take in the 2,000 calories a day he needed, but we felt we should let him try.

His doctor let us remove the nasogastric tube; but as we expected, Cyrus was too weak to eat 2,000 calories, and we had to replace the tube the next day. But we did so with Cyrus's consent—apparently he was satisfied that we'd at least given him a chance to try. From then on, he began eating more, and the jejunostomy tube wasn't necessary. A soft diet and 1,200 ml of Isocal supplied his nutritional needs, and Cyrus became strong enough to eat sitting up, which helped prevent reflux.

When Cyrus had been with us for 3 weeks, we began weaning him from the ventilator. The respiratory therapists, who'd helped him all along, encouraged him greatly. The first day, Cyrus spent an hour on the ventilator and an hour off. The second day, his time off was increased to 14 hours. He was doing well, even helping with the time-keeping. By the fourth day, he was up to 24 hours off, but secretions were becoming a problem. Cyrus began waving his skinny, accusing finger at the therapists if they were 2 minutes late in putting him back on the ventilator.

Once again, Cyrus became difficult. He refused to eat and even refused to sit up. His reply to every request was to shake his head "no."

What caused this abrupt change in Cyrus? It was easy to figure out. He'd probably realized what a long haul the weaning process would be and had gotten depressed. We told the doctor what we thought, and he decided to cut back on the time Cyrus spent off the ventilator until Cyrus seemed more ready to handle weaning. Physically, he was ready; all he needed was more self-confidence.

We continued to encourage him to express his feelings even though, at times, it was at our expense. Since he loved to complain about his food (the egg yolk was always too hard, the white too runny), we called the dietitian and asked if Cyrus could complain directly to her. She visited Cyrus, and we interpreted his pantomimes for her. After that, his meals improved.

We also knew Cyrus got angry when we made him comply with his physical therapy program. So one day when he refused to get out of bed to walk, we bargained that if he'd just walk to the door of his room, he could stick his tongue out at the nurse of his choice. He walked, stuck out his tongue, and chuckled all the way back to bed. Okay. So our ideas were a little unconventional. But they worked.

Our little extra attentions meant a lot to Cyrus. One particularly busy day we served him lunch at the nurses' station so one nurse could keep an eye on him and 16 monitors at the same time. To us, it was just a convenience. But Cyrus later told his wife that the nurses had let him "eat lunch with them" and that he'd felt honored.

As Cyrus regained confidence, his weaning progressed quickly. His nasogastric tube was removed, and after he'd been with us for 7 weeks, Cyrus made the final move himself. One night, he refused to use the ventilator. His doctor approved, and Cyrus was on his own. I don't think one of us breathed easily that night—except maybe Cyrus, who weaned himself without a bit of trouble.

The next day, Cyrus began a regimen of intermittent positive pressure breathing, and percussion followed by postural drainage. His sputum became more tenacious, and we increased his I.V. fluid intake.

Now that we knew he was on the road to recovery, we began laying the groundwork for his transfer out of our unit. To decrease his dependency on us, we assigned students and nurses he didn't know to care for him. At first, this annoyed him, and he insisted on knowing many of the newcomers' qualifications. We also arranged to have Cyrus's new nurses visit him so he'd feel more comfortable when he was moved.

Then the big day came: Cyrus's tracheostomy tube and I.V. were removed, and he was transferred out of our unit and onto a medical unit.

He remained in the hospital for another week, and we visited him whenever we could. He made rapid progress, and by the time of his discharge, he could sit up, bathe himself, feed himself, and walk 100 feet (3,000 cm) with assistance. He'd also gained 20 pounds (9 kg).

The day before Cyrus returned home, he visited our unit and gave us a huge, heart-shaped box of candy, saying, "This is for being so good to me." He also presented his physical and respiratory therapists with boxes of candy.

We were genuinely touched. Being good to Cyrus hadn't always been that easy, and some of our ways of dealing with his difficult behavior had been pretty unconventional to say the least. But they'd worked—they'd helped him vent his anger and feel more in control. And we were convinced they'd probably relieved tension by showing Cyrus that we weren't "all business," that we had a sense of humor too.

Of course, nursing *is* serious business. But sometimes a little humor and unconventionality are just what we need to reach a difficult patient.

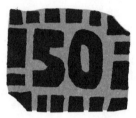

With So Little Hope, Michael Needed a Second Chance

MAUREEN O'BRIEN, RN

If there's one lesson ingrained in us in nursing school, it's to "go by the book." Yet how often in going by the book we blithely make assumptions about a patient that turn out to be quite wrong. I never had a better example of this than when I was a student nurse on a continuing care unit.

Assuming the worst for 25-year-old Michael Kennedy was easy. He'd been in a comatose state for 9 months, and his prognosis had hardly changed. One doctor's report summed up his bleak neurologic status: "persistent vegetative state from which recovery is not expected."

Coping with dehumanizing phrases like "persistent vegetative state" and the attitudes that go with them was only half my battle. While setting goals for Michael, I had to constantly weigh my own lack of nursing experience against my intuitive belief that he could be rehabilitated… against all clinical odds.

After a late-night card game, Michael, a salesman, had been found unconscious on his bathroom floor. He'd been rushed 100 miles (160 km) by an air ambulance to a Toronto hospital, where a computerized tomography scan revealed a large right subdural hematoma. To evacuate the hematoma, doctors performed a right craniotomy. Then, because of rising intracranial pressure, he was given a craniectomy and right temporal lobe decompression the next day.

A month later, still comatose, he was transferred to a hospital near his parents' home. At first he was on a medical unit, but after 4 months, when his level of awareness didn't improve, he was moved to the continuing care unit.

Up until this point, Michael had had no rehabilitation. His left side remained spastic and stiff; his right side, flaccid. He responded to pinpricks or loud noises with only a grimace and bilateral decorticate movement.

To help prevent his contractures, he was given passive range-of-motion (ROM) exercises. He also was given 100 mg phenytoin sodium (Dilantin) t.i.d. for prophylactic seizure control and 10 mg diazepam (Valium) t.i.d. for anxiety via a nasogastric tube. But other than tending to his basic needs, the medical staff hadn't started a coordinated rehabilitation program.

I met Michael when I was assigned to the unit

he was on. Lying on an air mattress with a tracheostomy, nasogastric tube, and indwelling catheter, he looked like a visual teaching aid from a neurology textbook. Six feet tall, with thin, auburn hair, Michael might've been considered handsome at one time. But weighing barely 130 pounds (58.5 kg) now, he looked pale and emaciated.

Feeling uneasy just standing there, I started to introduce myself. Suddenly Michael exhaled deeply. He was in a semi-Fowler's position with wrists flexed inward under his chin—typical decorticate posturing—and a clot of yellow mucus, expelled from his trach, shot across the room and splattered on the door beside me.

I jumped. The next thing I knew I was backing out of the doorway, hearing myself nervously saying, "Oh, I guess I'll see you a little later."

Fighting my own nervousness, I stopped by his room the next day for a proper introduction. I watched him closely. His facial features softened as I continued to talk in a clear, strong voice. His eyes were open, but they didn't focus—each pupil stared in a different direction. But looking into them, I realized that despite his poor prognosis, Michael seemed to have some dim awareness of his surroundings.

That afternoon I told my instructor that I wanted Michael to be my patient. Of course, making even a little progress with Michael would take an enormous amount of time—time that regular staff nurses didn't have to spend with one patient. But since I was a student nurse, my schedule was flexible, and Michael would be my only patient. What's more, despite my lack of clinical experience (or maybe *because* of it), I didn't have a head full of preconceived notions. I didn't believe Michael was a "human vegetable."

And neither did his parents. I met them the next day while I was administering Michael's 4 p.m. tube feeding of a dietary supplement. They visited their son twice a day, and over the next few days we got to know each other. I knew how important their support would be to Michael during the coming months.

So with my instructor's support, I started Michael's rehabilitation program. First of all, I performed passive ROM exercises on him every 3 hours, supplementing his regular once-a-day physical therapy program. At the same time, I played

tape recordings of soft, contemporary music he'd liked before he'd become comatose.

I spent as much time as I could just talking to him. I routinely explained who I was and what I was going to do before giving any nursing care, and I kept my sentences short and direct. I always tried to stand or sit where he could see me. His eyes showed me how afraid he was.

To help relax him and stimulate his awareness, I massaged his fingers with lotion every few hours. Usually he'd just hold my hand loosely. But by the end of the first week, his grasp could become viselike if I stopped or made a sudden movement to leave. Then his fingers would have to be pried loose, one at a time.

Some days, I spent as long as 8 hours with him, and all that attention paid off. His pupils were focusing now and he could shift his attention from my face to the face of someone just entering the room. I also realized that by talking to him comfortably, I could change his facial expressions and relax his entire body. Soon, Michael even began to relax during his ROM exercises, which caused him pain.

I paid particular attention to his appearance, asking his mother to split some of his favorite sport shirts down the back and sew on cloth ties so he wouldn't have to dress in hospital pajamas. I did this because I thought it would make him psychologically stronger for rehabilitation.

My second week as his nurse, I took him outside, with the hospital's cooperation. To transport a comatose patient like Michael, I needed a geriatric chair and an orderly's help to keep his tubes from tangling. With the support of my instructor, I got both.

It'd been nearly a year since Michael had not been surrounded by four walls. The wind blew on his face, and I watched as his eyes darted back and forth as a motorcycle started up suddenly. He was becoming more aware of the environment each day.

My optimism was renewed the next day, when with the head nurse's permission I plugged his trach tube and, to my surprise, Michael made throaty growling sounds as if he wanted to talk.

Once, Michael haltingly raised his left hand to pull out his nasogastric tube. Of course, I asked him not to do that. But secretly I was happy he'd attempted to fight the spasticity of his arm and to exert his own will.

His mother and I speculated about what his first words might be. "He'll probably tell one of us to shut up," Mrs. Kennedy joked.

A month had passed since Michael became my patient and, by being consistent and persistent, I'd helped raise his level of awareness. My next priority was to try to get his tubes removed. I felt that

 coping with dehumanizing phrases like "persistent vegetative state" and the attitudes that go with them was only half my battle. While setting goals for Michael, I constantly had to weigh my own lack of nursing experience against my intuitive belief that he could be rehabilitated... against all clinical odds.

his tracheostomy, nasogastric tube, and indwelling catheter all hindered his progress toward becoming more aware.

Oral feedings should be the first step, but I knew that as long as Michael received 2,000 calories primarily through nasogastric tube feedings, he'd never be interested in oral feedings. Besides, he had a great deal of trouble swallowing and I thought it was because of his nasogastric tube. I told his doctor what I thought, and a week later the nasogastric tube came out.

From that point on, Michael began getting six small meals a day rather than three large ones to avoid vomiting and aspiration. The dietitian recommended we start him on foods like yogurt and applesauce, then pureed meat and mashed potatoes. Just getting Michael to swallow was a tortuously long process, but with the constant encouragement of his mother, he began to gain weight.

Sometimes during his meals, Michael would assert his independence. He would raise his bib to his mouth with his left hand and spit his food into it, hoping none of us caught on. But early one evening while being fed, Michael seemed particularly vexed. He kept spitting out the food as fast as his mother could spoon it in. Frustrated, he suddenly growled, "Don't... want... any... more...." We were too stunned to answer him.

A week later, Michael spoke again. In a low, soft whisper, he asked me, "Why... am... I... here?" I explained what had happened to him and where he now was. He listened—or seemed to anyway—but didn't utter a sound when I answered his question. I made a point never to give him false hope by saying that he'd recover completely. Instead I said he was doing better each day.

During the next month, I started plugging his trach tube for progressively longer periods. When he continued to breathe comfortably, the doctor removed his trach tube altogether. This was an important step toward improving Michael's speech. With his tracheostomy removed, I hoped that he'd be able to talk more easily.

When Michael's catheter became plugged, it was removed. I asked his doctor if, instead of having the catheter reinserted, he could use a urinal. Michael was subsequently put on a urinal schedule, which he followed fairly closely.

I also asked his doctor to discontinue Michael's diazepam during the day. I felt the combination of diazepam and phenytoin sodium was unnecessarily tranquilizing. When the doctor agreed, I saw an increase in Michael's alertness during the next few days.

My next goal was to prepare him to visit his parents in their home. Once again with the co-operation of the hospital, I borrowed a high-backed wheelchair and accompanied Michael home in the hospital van. Later that day, after we'd returned to the hospital, he growled, "Want...to...go... home." There were tears in his eyes. I promised him that he would go home again soon.

Visiting home at least twice a week was important for Michael's emotional outlook. The visits gave him incentive. And they were rewarding in other ways, too. One evening he very slowly and messily ate corn-on-the-cob and drank a small glass of beer. To help him drink, I propped his left elbow on a cushion. Then, he slowly lowered his mouth to the glass. He'd never have expended that much energy for a mere glass of apple juice in the hospital.

Michael's level of alertness continued to improve. He'd say two or three sentences to me or his parents every day. With encouragement, he could now tell me how many brothers and sisters he had and point to his ears, nose, hair, and eyes when asked to.

Although Michael was making excellent progress, he still refused to speak to anyone else. That worried us, particularly when his doctor decided to have him reassessed for rehabilitation. A good assessment might mean he'd be moved off the maintenance care floor and into a rehabilitation program. But he'd have to *talk* with the rehabilitation specialist before that would happen.

When I explained this to Michael, he asked, "What...should...I...do?"

"Michael, you've got to start talking to other people in the hospital," I said.

Looking at me sadly, he replied, "I can't."

But the next day he did. An orderly was washing his hair and accidentally got suds in Michael's eyes. Michael shook his head and groaned. "What's the matter, don't you like water?" the orderly asked.

"Not...in...my eyes," Michael said.

When the time came, Michael responded to most of the rehabilitation specialist's questions. He felt that Michael would continue to improve, but that his progress would be slow.

That was good news, of course, and later that week, Michael was moved to the rehabilitation unit, which meant he'd be up and dressed every day. Sixteen weeks had passed since he'd been thought of as "a human vegetable." No one thought of him that way any more.

Of course, Michael's recovery continues to this day. He lives with his parents, and although he still has trouble with short-term memory and speech and with occasional bouts of depression, he gets stronger and more independent each day.

During one of my almost daily visits, Michael suddenly told me, "I...can't...just...lie...here... anymore." Startled, I looked at him. He was *serious*.

"Then what are you going to do, Michael?" I asked.

"Going...to...get...a...job," he replied firmly.

Was he being unrealistic? For sure...at least, for *now*. But perhaps after a long period of rehabilitation...perhaps. Well, why not?

Why not, indeed. My experience with Michael taught me that if I must assume *anything* about a patient, let it be the best—not the worst. I also learned to go by the book, by all means. But after caring for Michael, I'd never be afraid to write a few new lines in that book myself.

Sergeant Caulder Thought He Was a P.O.W. – We Played Along

DEE ALMAN, RN

We learn certain rules in nursing school that later on, we try to put into practice. One rule I learned was: When you're caring for a delusional patient, *never* agree with or get involved in his delusion. This guideline worked with every patient except one: Sergeant Jeffrey Caulder.

Sergeant Caulder was wheeled into our emergency room one night after his car had been rammed by a drunken driver. He had a crushed lower left leg, lacerations of the left thigh, simple fractures of the lower left arm bones, a ruptured spleen, a compression rupture of the descending colon, a left hemopneumothorax, and a crushing injury to the left side of his head. To make matters worse, he was in a coma.

Emergency surgery was done to remove the sergeant's spleen and repair his bowel, but because our hospital doesn't have a neurosurgeon, we couldn't do anything for his head injury. The doctors decided we should observe him closely and, if any neurological deterioration was noticed, transfer him to a hospital that had a neurosurgeon.

When Sergeant Caulder arrived in the intensive care unit, he was still comatose. His head turned and twisted constantly, but the rest of his body was immobile. Parts of his left parietal and temporal bones had been crushed in the accident. The left side of his head was slightly swollen when we first saw him, and it continued to swell for 18 hours. For the next week, until the bone slivers began to heal, the area around the sergeant's left ear felt like a rotten muskmelon.

Sergeant Caulder's doctor wanted us to turn his patient right-back-left every 2 hours. But he'd warned us that absolutely no pressure was allowed on the left, crushed side of the sergeant's skull. The first order made the second one impossible, we thought. But the doctor offered no suggestions—just follow his orders, he said.

Trying to turn Sergeant Caulder was only the first of many challenges. We turned him on his right side, and put bed pillows between his knees, and against his chest and back to hold him in position. When we turned him on his back, we applied tincture of benzoin to his forehead and chin, stuck Montgomery straps to the benzoin, and attached a 10-pound sandbag to the right side strap openings with Montgomery ties. The sandbag held the sergeant's head upright, so he couldn't turn to the left.

Then we spent a frantic 2 hours figuring out how to turn him on his left side. Somehow (necessity *is* the mother of invention) we came up with a solution. First, we removed the sandbag. Then we took a doughnut-shaped foam-rubber cushion, and using the Montgomery ties again, tied the foam to the left side of his head. The crushed area fit perfectly inside the doughnut hole, and the sergeant's head was both elevated and cushioned. Again, we used pillows to hold him in place.

On the sergeant's third day in the intensive care unit (ICU), his left arm twitched—meaning one of two things. He was either coming out of his coma, or he was about to have a seizure. But the sergeant wasn't having a seizure, because the next thing he did was pull at his Foley catheter. When we gently removed his left hand from the Foley, he grabbed for his nasogastric tube.

We did the only thing we could—we loosely restrained his left arm. But when the sergeant discovered he couldn't move his arm, he went wild, dragging the sandbag around the top of his bed.

Thinking fast, we released his arm, but taped his nasogastric tube down the right side of his face. We taped the urinary drainage tube to his immobile right leg and snapped a pair of orthopedic pajama bottoms on backwards so he couldn't pull out the Foley. The sergeant picked unsuccessfully at the tape on his cheek, but he left the tubes alone.

On the fourth day after his surgery, the sergeant's left leg twitched. We were busy with other patients, but the thud of his cast hitting the floor was unmistakable. When we reached the sergeant's bed, his left leg was on the floor. How he managed to squeeze his leg, cast and all, under the padded side rail, was anybody's guess. But Sergeant Caulder was full of surprises, as we were soon to find out.

"I have to go to the bathroom," he said. And, with one leg already on the floor, he seemed to be on his way. We restored him to bed, and then we told him about his accident, his injuries, and oriented him to time and place. He said he didn't remember the accident at all, but we assured him that temporary amnesia after a traumatic event wasn't uncommon.

"I guess I was unconscious when they captured me," he said. *He's just confused,* we thought.

But he was more than confused. Poor Mrs. Chang, the Oriental housekeeper, was the first target of Sergeant Caulder's delusion. When she entered his room the next day, he threw a barrage of curses and a roll of tape at her.

When we arrived, the sergeant was livid with rage. "That guard just threatened me!" he shouted. When we told him she was the house–keeper, he snapped: "Don't try to trick me, I know this is a Korean prisoner-of-war camp. Whose side are you on, mine or theirs?"

We realized then what we were up against—a full-blown delusion. Of course we were on his side, we told him. Hadn't we cared for him while he was unconscious?

Sergeant Caulder seemed to accept our words, because he smiled complacently and nodded. What we didn't yet realize was that he'd already worked us into his delusion—we were captured medics.

We hoped that by keeping all Oriental personnel out of his room, we could avoid another scene, so we wrote a note to this effect in his care plan. We also posted a "Keep out—inquire at desk" sign on his door. But things weren't that simple.

The next person who entered the sergeant's room was the social worker. She was greeted by a patient who cringed and snapped obscenities when she tried to touch him. The sergeant had apparently divided everyone in the hospital into "us" and "them," with all strangers being "them."

We nurses in the "us" category (the ones who'd been at the sergeant's bedside after his confrontation with the housekeeper) began to introduce him to everyone involved in his care. When we introduced the sergeant's doctor to his own patient, the doctor immediately ordered a psychiatric consult.

That evening, the staff psychiatrist visited Sergeant Caulder. We were *not* to agree with his delusion, the doctor decided. If the sergeant insisted someone was a prison guard we should simply tell him the person's name and job. The psychiatrist was confident his idea would work. We had a more than sneaking suspicion it wouldn't.

For the next 24 hours, we followed the psychiatrist's suggestions. The sergeant continued to insist it was 1952 and he was a prisoner of war (POW). We couldn't convince him there weren't Korean guards out there somewhere.

Our relationship with the sergeant deteriorated rapidly. The idea that we were "turncoats" resurfaced. When we tried to touch him, he cursed and fought us. He needed so much care, but it was becoming impossible to give him that care. So we called the psychiatrist again. After he visited the sergeant a second time, he agreed with us—we'd have to accept the delusion. If we didn't, and the sergeant continued to reject our care, he might die.

So we stopped disagreeing with the sergeant, although we never actually said, "You're right, we're all POWs." We weren't wild about being actors in his delusion, but fighting him every step of the way hadn't worked either. Now that he accepted us again, his care should've been easier, but we ran into other problems.

On his 11th day in the ICU, the sergeant passed flatus, so his nasogastric tube was removed, and oral fluids were ordered. I was there to give him his first glass of water.

"I'm not drinking that," he said. "They've drugged it so I'll talk." I poured some of the water into a medicine cup, drank a sip, and asked him if he'd drink *now*. He agreed.

Then I realized I'd forgotten to bring a drinking straw. Not wanting to leave the room while he was still cooperative, I attempted to help him drink from the glass. I elevated the head of his bed, walked around to his right side, and began to tip the glass toward his mouth. Shrieking, he knocked the glass from my hand.

Now what? I thought, as I ran to the foot of the bed to clean up the mess. "Where'd you go?" the sergeant said, wild-eyed. "While you were gone, a guard sneaked up and tried to poison me."

Then it dawned on me what had happened. We retested the sergeant's eyes, and discovered that the entire right side of his visual field was missing. When we stood on his right side, we vanished. We couldn't do anything to correct his vision, but we could make sure we only approached him from his left side. So we all became temporarily left-handed.

The next day, as I clumsily tried to give him a glass of orange juice, his left hand closed around mine. All his movements up to this point had been erratic, but this was a purposeful movement. He obviously wanted to feed himself. He spilled most of his juice the first few times, but we covered the top of his unbreakable glass with plastic wrap and poked a straw through the plastic. Soon the sergeant was taking all liquids with very few spills.

Although the sergeant was regaining control of his left side, we sensed something was wrong elsewhere. He still had a low-grade fever, and was still on I.V. antibiotic therapy.

We sensed he was in pain, but he refused to complain. Complaining was unmanly, he said, considering the torture the other POWs were undergoing. He'd heard them screaming during the night. (What he'd actually heard was another patient crying.)

When your patient won't admit he's in pain, you have to rely on other resources to discover where the pain is, and how severe it is. We checked regularly for elevated pulse and blood pressure, and watched to see if he was sweating. He finally gave us a signal that he was in pain—a facial tic in his right temple seemed to occur when the pain was severe.

Two days later, the sergeant complained of pain for the first time. "They" were stabbing his left shoulder. A chest X-ray revealed a fully expanded lung and a dense shadow just below his diaphragm. The sergeant had a subdiaphragmatic abscess.

He needed immediate surgery, and we knew we had a problem on our hands. We had to move him out of his room, where he felt relatively secure, to where "they" were. Since we knew we'd never get him out of the room while he was conscious, the doctor anesthetized him in his bed, by injecting sodium pentothal into his I.V. line.

The abscess was drained successfully, and we acted as recovery room nurses, knowing he'd be terrified if he awoke with a group of strangers staring down at him. We never told the sergeant about his surgery.

On the sergeant's 30th day in the ICU, his doctor decided it was time to transfer his patient to a general surgical ward. How we'd move him from the ICU to the ward was, of course, *our* problem.

Preparing for the sergeant's transfer was like planning the Berlin airlift. First, we assured him that the new staff he'd meet were on "our" side. For the next 3 days, we introduced the entire surgical ward staff to the sergeant, coaching them beforehand.

What followed was probably the longest room-to-room transfer in hospital history. Moving Sergeant Caulder from his room to the ward took 3 days. Slowly, we pushed his bed out of the room, into the hall, to the nurses' station, to the hall outside the ward, and finally into the ward. One of us stayed with him all the time, giving him the same care we'd given him in his room, and introducing any strangers who walked by.

Sergeant Caulder had been our patient for 33 days. After his transfer, we'd stop to see him. Other than his continuing delusion, he seemed to be progressing, and he was always happy to see us. As we got busy with other patients, though, the time between our visits lengthened. One day I stopped by, only to learn that he'd been discharged. Discharged into enemy teritory? No.

One night, 3 weeks after he'd left the ICU, Sergeant Caulder went to sleep a prisoner of war in Korea, and, inexplicably, awoke the next morning a patient in a U.S. Army hospital. The 7 weeks between his accident and his recovery from his delusion were a complete blank.

Three months after his discharge, the sergeant, accompanied by his psychiatrist, visited us. The sergeant was thin, pale, and limping on his left side. His head was still slightly swollen, giving him a lopsided appearance. But he looked just fine to us.

"The doctor says you were great to me while I was here," he said. "I'm sorry I can't remember any of you. Guess it's that darned accident amnesia."

Darned accident amnesia? We were amazed. Then, as the sergeant walked around the rest of the unit, the doctor took us aside. "I haven't told him about his delusion, and I'd appreciate it if you wouldn't tell him, either. He'd be mighty embarrassed if he ever knew what a damned fool he made of himself."

But we didn't think he'd made a fool of himself. He'd given us an experience we'd never forget. They say "The worst deluded are the self–deluded," and we'd have been deluding ourselves if we'd tried to follow the old rules with Sergeant Caulder. But we all agreed on one thing—the sergeant couldn't have chosen a better time period to erase.

Index

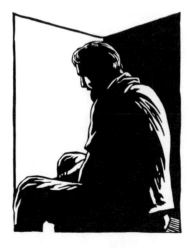

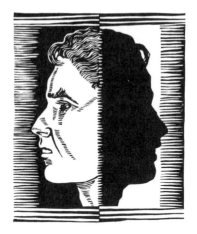